Legal Aspects
of Speech-Language
Pathology
and Audiology

Legal Aspects
of Speech-Language
Pathology
and Audiology

FRANKLIN H. SILVERMAN
Marquette University/Medical College of Wisconsin

Legal Aspects of Speech-Language Pathology and Audiology

an overview of law for clinicians, researchers, and teachers

PRENTICE-HALL, INC., Englewood Cliffs, New Jersey 07632

Library of Congress Cataloging in Publication Data

Silverman, Franklin H. (date)
    Legal aspects of speech-language pathology and audiology.

    Includes bibliographies and indexes.
    1. Speech therapists—Legal status, laws, etc.
—United States. 2. Audiologists—Legal status, laws, etc.—United States. I. Title.
KF2915.S63S53 1983   344.73'041   82-11280
ISBN 0-13-528109-1   347.30441

Editorial/production supervision by Linda Benson
Cover design by Edsal Enterprises
Manufacturing buyers: Edmund W. Leone and Ron Chapman

©1983 by Prentice-Hall, Inc., Englewood Cliffs, N.J. 07632

All rights reserved. No part of this book
may be reproduced in any form or
by any means without permission in writing
from the publisher.

Printed in the United States of America

10 9 8 7 6 5 4 3 2 1

ISBN 0-13-528109-1

PRENTICE-HALL INTERNATIONAL, INC., *London*
PRENTICE-HALL OF AUSTRALIA PTY. LIMITED, *Sydney*
EDITORA PRENTICE-HALL DO BRAZIL, Ltda., *Rio de Janeiro*
PRENTICE-HALL CANADA INC., *Toronto*
PRENTICE-HALL OF INDIA PRIVATE LIMITED, *New Delhi*
PRENTICE-HALL OF JAPAN, INC., *Tokyo*
PRENTICE-HALL OF SOUTHEAST ASIA PTE. LTD., *Singapore*
WHITEHALL BOOKS LIMITED, WELLINGTON, *New Zealand*

To speech-language pathologists and audiologists who use the law to promote the welfare of the persons they serve professionally

Contents

Preface xi

1
Relevance of Law for the Speech-Language Pathologist and Audiologist 1

    Some Intersects Between Law, Professional Ethics, and Clinical Practice and Research 3
    References 7

2
Our Legal System: An Overview of Professionally Relevant Aspects 9

    What Are Laws? 10
    Why Are Laws Obeyed? 11
    From What Sources Do Our Laws Originate? 18
    How Are the Laws That Make Up Our Legal System Categorized? 35
    How Are the Laws That Make Up Our Legal System Enforced? 37
    References 60

3
Licensure, Certification, Registration, and Accreditation 61

    What Is the Motivation for Initiating Licensure, Certification, Registration, and Accreditation? 62

viii Contents

    How Are Occupations Regulated? 65
    What Approaches Have Been Used to Regulate the Practice of Speech-
        Language Pathology and Audiology? 73
    How Can Certification, Accreditation, Licensure, or Registration Be Lost? 74
    Procedures Used for Taking Away Certification, Accreditation, Licensure,
        and Registration 76
    References 77

4
Contractual Obligations to Clients and Others 78

    Events That Can Result in the Creation of a Contract 79
    Contractual Aspects of the Client-Clinician Relationship 90
    References 91

5
Professional Ethics and Law 92

    Relationship Between Ethics and Law 93
    Ethics and the Clinician 95
    Code of Ethics of the American Speech-Language-Hearing Association 104
    References 106

6
Malpractice and Other Torts 108

    What Is a Tort? 109
    Types of Torts 111
    Tort Litigation and the Speech-Language Pathologist and Audiologist 121
    References 121

7
Records Management 122

    Kinds of Data Regarded by the Courts as Being Part of a Clinic Record 123
    Some Aspects of Clinical Records Management on Which There Are Legal
        Restrictions 123
    References 128

8
Implications of Copyright and Patent Law for the Practitioner and Teacher 129

    Objectives of Copyright and Patent Law 129
    Provisions of the Copyright Act of 1976 131
    Provisions of U.S. Patent Law 136
    References 139

9
Legal Aspects of Administration and Private Practice   140

    Organizational Structures for Clinical Facilities   *140*
    Legal Aspects of the Employer-Employee Relationship   *143*
    Advertising   *147*
    Record Keeping for Tax and Other Business Purposes   *147*
    Addendum   *148*
    References   *148*

10
Legal and Ethical Considerations in Clinical Research   149

    Need for Protecting Research Subjects   *149*
    Informed Consent as a Vehicle for Protecting Investigators and Institutions from Tort Litigation   *152*
    Legal-Ethical Implications of the Therapeutic-Nontherapeutic Continuum in Clinical Research   *153*
    Documenting a Person's Informed Consent to Serve as *a Research Subject*   *160*
    References   *160*

11
Serving as an Expert Witness   161

    Subjects About Which Speech-Language Pathologists and Audiologists Have Testified as Expert Witnesses   *162*
    Functioning as an Expert Witness   *164*
    The Expert Witness Fee   *171*
    References   *171*

12
Lobbying for Legislative Change   173

    What Is a Lobbyist?   *174*
    Approaches Used by Lobbyists to Influence Legislators   *175*
    Functioning as a Lobbyist   *178*
    Playing an Advocacy Role   *179*
    References   *180*

Appendix A
Representative Release Forms   181

Appendix B
Representative Regulations Governing the Use of Human Subjects   187

Appendix C
Selected Legislation Relevant to Speech-Language Pathologists and Audiologists 191

Appendix D
Constitution of the United States 193

Appendix E
Selected Ethical Codes of the American Speech-Language-Hearing Association 1930-1979 209

Glossary of Legal Terms 217

Index 221

Preface

The clinical functioning of speech-language pathologists and audiologists at any given time is determined not only by their clinical skills and the needs of their clients, but also by *numerous legal-ethical restrictions and obligations.* These come from a number of sources: the Constitution; municipal, state, and federal legislation; regulations from state and federal administrative agencies; legal precedents derived from court decisions (i.e., common law); and professional codes of ethics. Speech-language pathologists and audiologists must be aware of the legal-ethical restrictions and obligations that they are required by law to consider in their relationships with their clients and their families; with employees, and employers, and other professionals; with state and federal government agencies; and with all others with whom they interact professionally. Ignorance of the law unfortunately does not protect one from the consequences of violating it!

This book deals with legal-ethical issues that impinge on clinical practice and research in speech-language pathology and audiology. My primary objective is to provide clinicians and investigators with the basic information they need to use the law to promote the welfare of those whom they serve professionally. *This book is not intended to serve as a substitute for legal consultation.* Rather, it is meant to *enhance* such consultation by providing readers with the intuitive understanding of legal concepts that they need to formulate questions that will yield desired information and to interpret the answers given.

Legal Aspects of Speech-Language Pathology and Audiology is divided into two parts. The first part (Chapters 1 and 2) provides basic information about how

xii   *Preface*

the law impinges on clinical practice and research and how the legal system functions. The second part (Chapters 3 through 12) provides information about how specific aspects of law can be applied to promote the welfare of those whom speech-language pathologists and audiologists serve professionally.

The book contains a set of representative release forms (Appendix A); the Nuremberg Code and the Declaration of Helsinki, both of which deal with the use of human subjects in research (Appendix B); a listing of legislation relevant to speech-language pathologists and audiologists (Appendix C); the Constitution of the United States (Appendix D); selected ethical codes of the American Speech-Language-Hearing Association, 1930-1979 (Appendix E); and a glossary of legal terms.

It is impossible to give credit to the many sources from which the concepts presented in this book have been drawn. The book is the result of years of reading and hundreds of hours of conversation with students and colleagues in the areas of speech-language pathology, audiology, and law. Thus, I cannot credit this or that concept to a specific person, but I can say thank you to all who have helped, particularly my graduate students at Marquette University, whose questions and criticisms through the years have helped me to clarify my own ideas.

Special thanks are due to the American Speech-Language-Hearing Association for giving me the opportunity to serve as the first Wisconsin Coordinator for its Congressional Action Contact Network. It was this experience that was primarily responsible for my developing a strong interest in legal aspects of speech-language pathology and audiology. Some special thanks also are due to the following persons for their helpful reviews of the book proposal, the completed manuscript, or both: Dr. Daniel Boone, University of Arizona; Dr. Melvin Cohen, Loma Linda University; Dr. Richard Flower, University of California; Attorney Diane Mashie, Washington, D.C.; and Attorney Philip Padden, Milwaukee, Wisconsin.

Franklin H. Silverman

Legal Aspects
of Speech-Language
Pathology
and Audiology

1

Relevance of Law for the Speech-Language Pathologist and Audiologist

The clinical functioning of speech-language pathologists and audiologists at any given moment is determined not only by their clinical skills and the needs of their clients but also by numerous *legal-ethical restraints and obligations.* These originate from a number of sources, including the Constitution; municipal, state, and federal legislation; regulations from state and federal administrative agencies (such as state and federal departments of education); legal precedent derived from court decisions (known as *common law*); and professional codes of ethics. Failure to consider these restraints and obligations adequately when functioning clinically can result in such consequences as being fired by one's employer; being sued by a client or a client's family; not being reimbursed by a private, state, or federal "insurance agency" for services provided; loss of certification or licensure; and having one's clients not receive services to which they are or should be entitled by law. It is crucial, therefore, that speech-language pathologists and audiologists be aware of the legal-ethical restraints and obligations that they are required by law to consider in their relationships with their clients and their families, employers, employees, other professionals, state and federal government agencies, and others with whom they interact professionally.

The primary objective of this chapter is to heighten your awareness of the legal-ethical restraints and obligations that influence your functioning as a clinician, clinical researcher, or clinician-investigator (for a discussion of the clinician-investigator concept see Chapter 2 of Silverman, 1977). I will attempt to achieve this objective by describing the intersect (i.e., area of overlap) between law, pro-

occurred in both instances would be *malpractice.* A claimed injury to the *reputation* or *feelings* of a plaintiff who is a professional could occur if a speech-language pathologist or audiologist *orally* indicated to potential clients that the professional was unethical or incompetent (tort of slander). If the reference was made in *writing,* the tort would be that of *libel.*

The "Unwritten" Contract Inherent in the Client-Clinician Relationship

The relationship between client and clinician is governed, in part, by *contract law* (Corbin, 1952). When a clinician offers to provide therapy for a client and the client (or someone legally responsible for him or her) accepts the offer, a contract may be formed between them. Contracts need not be written to be legally enforceable. Problems develop when the terms of the contract—that is, the obligations that both parties assume under it—are not fully understood by both parties. A client, for example, may assume that by offering therapy a clinician is indicating an ability to cure a particular communicative disorder. If the clinician fails to cure it, the client may regard the contract as having been *breached* and refuse to pay for some or all of the clinician's services. A clinician who had some knowledge of contract law probably could prevent such misunderstandings.

Serving as an Expert Witness

Speech-language pathologists and audiologists are asked to testify as experts in their fields in both federal and state courts and administrative hearings (such as those associated with the implementation of P.L. 94-142, which mandates that school districts meet the educational needs of all handicapped children for whom they are responsible). They may serve in this role at the request of the plaintiff or defendant in a case that is to be heard by a court or of any of the parties involved in an administrative hearing. A speech-language pathologist, for example, may be asked to testify about the competency of an aphasic to continue to manage his or her financial affairs; an audiologist may be asked to testify about the status of a plaintiff's hearing in a worker's compensation case.

Lobbying for Legislation Beneficial to the Communicatively Handicapped and the Profession

Since the providing of clinical services and the conduct of research is regulated by both state and federal legislation, speech-language pathologists and audiologists should have some interest in encouraging legislators at both state and federal levels to support bills that would benefit the communicatively handicapped and the profession and to amend or not support bills that could be detrimental to either or both. They can do this by informing their representatives specifically why they feel it would be in society's best interest if a particular bill were supported, amended, or voted down. By assuming this responsibility they increase the probability that their legislators will consider the issues they have raised when deciding how to vote on the bill. Most senators and representatives appreciate such lobbying because it helps them cast more informed votes. Some speech-language pathologists and audiologists devote much time to lobbying through participation in the Congressional Action Contact Network of the American Speech-Language-Hearing Association (Dowling, 1973) and those of some state speech and hearing associations that have been modeled after it.

Serving as an Advocate for Clients

Speech-language pathologists and audiologists have a responsibility to ensure that their clients receive the services to which they are entitled by law. To assume this responsiblity they must be aware of federal and state statutes that could facilitate the delivery of services to their clients, for example, by providing complete or partial funding. (Relevant statutes or parts thereof include Medicare and P.L. 94-142.) In some cases they can play this advocacy role merely by making a client or a client's family aware of such statutes and explaining how to apply for services under them. In other cases speech-language pathologists and audiologists serve as *intermediaries* between the client or family and the state or federal agency from whom assistance is being sought by providing the agency with information about the client or indicating to an agency why the client appears to be entitled to certain services. Speech-language pathologists and audiologists may also have to serve as advocates for reasons unrelated to their clients' communicative behaviors. A speech-language pathologist employed in a school, for example, may have to assume an advocacy role for a client who appears to be a "battered child" (O'Toole, 1974).

Clinical Records Management

Speech-language pathologists and audiologists, regardless of the setting in which they work, are required to maintain records on their clients. Management of such records has legal-ethical considerations. The confidentiality of the information in them must be maintained, and at the same time it must be possible to release specific information in them to other professionals or agencies when a client or client's family request. Also, they must be maintained in such a manner that the client's *freedom of access* to them (which is mandated by law) is unlikely to be detrimental to either client or clinician. Another important consideration concerns *subpoena* procedures: what must be released under various circumstances, the rights of the client in such instances, and monitoring record entries with a view to the possibility of subpoena.

Copyright and Patent Law

Speech-language pathologists and audiologists are both consumers and producers of copyrighted and patented materials and apparatus. There are legal restrictions on how they can utilize and reproduce such materials and apparatus for clinical, educational, and research purposes. Some such restrictions are imposed by the Copyright Act of 1976. Under this act, all materials developed by or for clinicians are *automatically* protected by copyright, regardless of whether they have been distributed commercially or have been formally copyrighted.

Administering a Clinical Program

Speech-language pathologists and audiologists (whether in private practice or in a school, hospital, or other clinical setting) are often called on to function as administrators, a role with legal-ethical aspects. When hiring employees (at both professional and clerical levels), for example, they must comply with federal regulations prohibiting discrimination against women, minorities, and the handicapped. They also must be in compliance with federal regulations when developing and managing a clinical record system. In addition, they must be aware of ethical considerations when deciding how to make the public aware of clinical services. These are only a few of the legal-ethical restrictions and obligations that the administrator of a clinical program must consider.

Establishing a Private Practice

A number of legal-ethical considerations arise when establishing a part-time or full-time private practice, many of which were mentioned in the preceding section on administering a clinical program. In addition, since a private practice is a *small business,* state and federal regulations for establishing and operating such businesses must be followed. A legal structure for the practice must be selected—should it be set up as a proprietorship, partnership, or corporation? (Some professionals in private practice incorporate in order to reduce their personal financial liability if they should be unsuccessful.) Also, a bookkeeping system that is adequate for tax and other purposes must be established.

Licensure and Certification

Legal-ethical restrictions on clinical practice in speech-language pathology and audiology are imposed by state licensure laws and American Speech-Language-Hearing Association certification. Every state, through a department that oversees public instruction, credentials speech-language pathologists who wish to work in its public schools. Some states also license speech-language pathologists and audiologists who do not work in the schools. The academic requirements for state licensure as a speech-language pathologist or audiologist tend to be quite similar to those for the certificates of clinical competence in speech-language pathology and audiology awarded by the American Speech-Language-Hearing Association.

Ethical Considerations in Clinical Practice and Research

Speech-language pathologists and audiologists, like the members of all professions, are required to function in a manner consistent with a code (or codes) of professional ethics and a "higher" ethical code, that of the society in which they function. The American Speech-Language-Hearing Association has a code of ethics (Code of Ethics of the American Speech and Hearing Association, 1979) and some state speech and hearing associations also have such codes. These codes include both restraints and obligations on clinical practice in speech-language pathology and audiology. They typically place restrictions on advertising and oblige practitioners to refer their clients to other professionals (physicians, dentists, other speech language pathologists or audiologists, etc.) when such referrals would appear to be in the best interest of their clients. These codes also place restraints on the activities of the clinical researcher, particularly with regard to protecting the person, reputation, and feelings of subjects. The professional activities of practitioners and researchers also are influenced by "higher" ethical codes. One such code that would influence the functioning of both these groups in the United States is *Judeo-Christian ethics.* An aspect of this code that is relevant clinically is referred to in the bioethics literature as the *ethics of manipulation* (Häring, 1975). This deals with ethical considerations when planning how to manipulate or control the behavior of a client or patient.

Legal Considerations in Clinical Research

In the design, conduct, and communication of research, an investigator must consider a number of legal-ethical restrictions and obligations. Most are intended to protect the person, reputation, and feelings of research subjects. Investigators, for example, must be able to document that they have obtained the *informed consent* of the persons who are to serve as subjects in their studies (Freund, 1970). For their consent to be *informed,* subjects must be made aware of any possible adverse effects they could experience as a result of participation in the research. Investigators are also required to protect subjects from harm to their reputations and feelings when reporting the results of their research, either keeping the identities of subjects unrecognizable or obtaining an appropriate release from them. Obtaining a release is particularly important when still photographs, motion pictures, audiotapes, or videotapes of the subjects are used as a part of a presentation of the research findings. (A form that can be used for this purpose is included in Appendix A.)

REFERENCES

Code of Ethics of the American Speech and Hearing Association, 1979. *Asha,* 21, 25-26 (1979).

CORBIN, A. L., *Corbin on Contracts.* St. Paul, Minn.: West Publishing Company (1952).

DOWLING, R. J., *ASHA Handbook for Congressional Action Contacts.* Washington, D.C.: American Speech and Hearing Association (1973).

FREUND, P. (Ed.), *Experimentation with Human Subjects.* New York: George Braziller (1970).

HÄRING, B., *Ethics of Manipulation.* New York: Seabury Press (1975).

O'TOOLE, T. J., The speech clinician and child abuse. *Language, Speech, and Hearing Services in Schools*, 5, 103-106 (1974).

PROSSER, W. L., *Law of Torts* (4th Ed.). St. Paul, Minn.: West Publishing Company (1971).

SILVERMAN, F. H., *Research Design in Speech Pathology and Audiology*. Englewood Cliffs, N.J.: Prentice-Hall (1977).

2

Our Legal System: An Overview of Professionally Relevant Aspects

In the preceding chapter we briefly considered some of the impacts our legal system has on clinical practice and research in speech-language pathology and audiology. Before exploring such impacts in greater depth, we shall consider the overall structure of our legal system, with particular emphasis on those aspects that are important for understanding the intersect beteweeen law and clinical practice and research (see Figure 1-1).

We begin by defining law through a consideration of its impacts on interpersonal relationships. Our entire system of law can be viewed as being motivated by a desire to control or regulate aspects of the various types of interpersonal relationships in which persons participate in our society.

Next, we consider sources from which laws that seek to influence aspects of our interpersonal relationships arise. We will consider courts (common law), legislatures (federal, state, and municipal statutes), administrative agencies (regulations from state and federal departments and offices), and professional organizations (e.g., regulations from the American Speech-Language-Hearing Association concerning clinical certification).

Next, we describe the internal structure of our legal system, including the types, or categories, of law contained in it. This will include a discussion of the distinctions among (1) criminal, administrative, and civil law, (2) substantive and procedural law, and (3) common law and legislative statutes. Finally, we consider the mechanisms used for *enforcing* laws, with particular emphasis on the civil suit and the administrative hearing.

WHAT ARE LAWS?

Laws are rules courts will enforce that are intended to govern our interpersonal relationships. They place *restrictions* and *obligations* on our relationships with others. Failure to obey them is ordinarily *supposed* to result in some sort of penalty.

Laws, viewed as rules intended for governing interpersonal relationships, vary on several dimensions (aside from specific content), including:

1. *The number of persons to which they are applicable.* Regulations from the Wisconsin Department of Public Instruction concerning maximum and minimum sizes for public school speech-language pathologists' caseloads are applicable to fewer persons than regulations arising from a federal statute such as P.L. 94-142 (see Appendix C).

2. *Their relative strength.* Some laws are viewed as stronger, or more important, than others in the sense that some have *precedence* over others. If two laws of unequal strength are applicable to a specific situation, the stronger usually will prevail. If the regulations from a state department of public instruction indicated that school districts could be reimbursed for speech-language pathology services only for children whose communicative disorder is "educationally significant" and if a federal statute indicated that the criterion of educational significance could not be used to deny funding for such services, the federal statute would probably prevail because federal statutes usually have precedence over state statutes when both apply to the same situation.

3. *Their source.* The rules, or laws, that regulate our interpersonal relationships as speech-language pathologists or audiologists arise from a number of sources, including municipal, state, and federal legislation; state and federal constitutions; precedents from court decisions; regulations from state and federal administrative agencies; professional codes of ethics (such as those of the American Speech-Language-Hearing Association and of state speech and hearing associations); and regulations established by employers. While an employer's regulations are usually not thought of as "laws," they function as such in that one is expected to obey them or pay the penalty (e.g., receive a reprimand or be fired). Also, they are implicitly recognized as laws by the courts since they must be consistent with municipal, state, and federal laws. If, for example, an employer made a regulation that members of certain minority groups could not be hired, this regulation probably would be declared illegal by the courts (if they were asked to rule on it) because state and federal legislation, which would have precedence over employers' regulations, prohibits discrimination in hiring. Sources of laws are considered in greater depth elsewhere in this chapter.

4. *Their duration.* Some laws remain in effect only for a specified period of time; others remain in effect until some action is taken to change or terminate them. As a result of sunset laws, some state licensure boards for speech-language pathologists and audiologists terminate after a specific number of years unless the legislation that created them is reenacted by the legislature (Downey, 1979).

5. *Their degree of specificity.* The restrictions and obligations mandated by some laws are presented at a lower level of abstraction than they are for others. They are specified in greater detail. The two quotations that follow illustrate this dimension. They are from the laws of two states pertaining to minimum requirements for facilities for providing speech, language, and hearing therapy in the public schools.

> The school system shall provide a classroom of suitable size, in a distraction free area as required by the type of program or services to be established, with appropriate furniture, materials, supplies and equipment to meet the needs of the class or individual children to be served.
>
> For speech and hearing therapy services, a quiet, adequately lighted and ventilated room with an electrical outlet must be provided in each center for the exclusive use of the speech, language, and hearing therapist, during the times scheduled at the center.
>
> The space in each center must have one table with five medium size chairs, one teacher's chair, one bulletin board, one permanent or portable chalkboard, and one large mirror mounted so that the therapist and student may sit before it. (Digest of State Laws and Regulations for School Language, Speech, and Hearing Programs, 1973)

Obviously, the degree of specificity is greater (and the level of abstraction is lower) for the second than it is for the first.

6. *The probability that they will be obeyed.* Some laws (regulations) are more likely to be obeyed than are others. A law may not be obeyed because the restrictions or obligations that it imposes are contrary to the desires of the majority of the people to whom it applies (e.g., the "prohibition" amendment to the Constitution). Or a law may not be obeyed because it is viewed as inconsistent with natural law—that is, what one considers "right" or "fair." (Some people avoided the draft during the Vietnam War because they considered the war to be "wrong.") Finally, some people may not obey a law because the restrictions or obligations imposed by it are contrary to their desires, and they are willing to risk receiving a penalty for not obeying it.

WHY ARE LAWS OBEYED?

Our willingness (or lack of willingness) to obey the laws that make up our legal system can be *rationalized,* or explained, by certain philosophies (or principles) in which we believe. Representative ones are summarized in Figure 2-1. We utilize such philosophies (whether or not we are consciously aware of doing so) when deciding the extent to which we are willing to accept particular restrictions and obligations in our interpersonal relationships.

The philosophies included in Figure 2-1, which are those that appear to exert the greatest influence on our behavior, will be described briefly. (For further in-

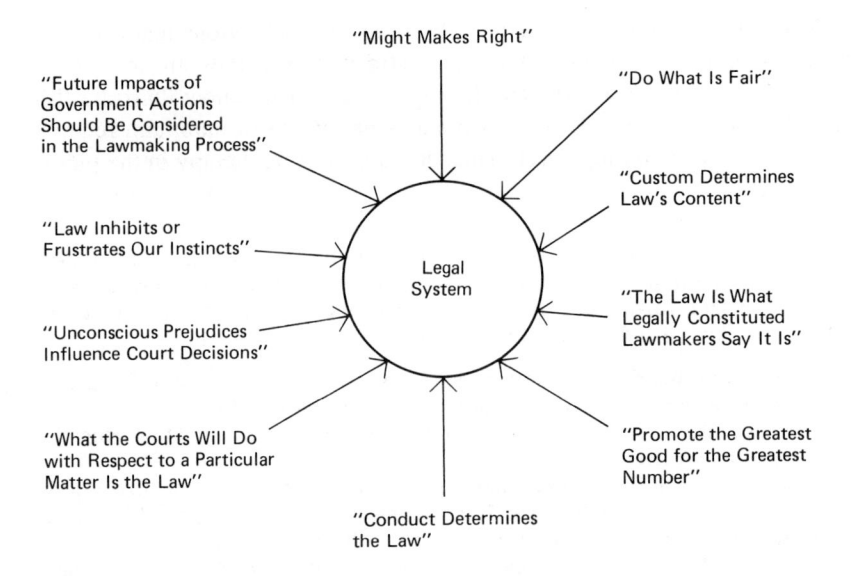

FIGURE 2-1 Some philosophies that have influenced (and are influencing) our legal system.

formation about them see Fisher, 1977, pp. 2-25, which was the primary source for this discussion.)

"Might Makes Right"

This philosophy suggests that we may accept restrictions and obligations because we view the source requesting us to do so as stronger than ourselves. The source can be one person (such as a supervisor) or a group of people (such as a state department of education). Its pronouncements (laws) can be communicated to us orally or in written form. Their impact on our interpersonal relationships can be either desirable or undesirable. The main point is that we do what we are asked to do because we regard the person or persons making the request as having the authority, or power, to do so. We are "following orders." Some clinicians (particularly student clinicians) accept supervisors' recommendations on this basis.

"Do What Is Fair"

This philosophy suggests that we have an obligation in our interpersonal relationships to do what is "right," "fair," "just," and "ethical." It further suggests that we are obliged to not do what is "wrong," "unfair," "unjust," and "unethical" *even if it is required by human laws.* This philosophy, known as *natural law,* is an aspect of our Judeo-Christian tradition. It assumes the existence of certain values that are so self-evident (perhaps God-given) that if laws formulated by humans are in conflict with them they should not be obeyed. Following World War II the

Nuremberg trials of Nazis for their murder of millions of Jews and Gypsies were justified on the basis of a breach of natural law. (There were no international laws at that time prohibiting genocide.) When we use our *conscience* as a guide for determining our behavior, we are functioning on the basis of natural law. Violating such law results in *guilt* feelings. Natural law, of course, is the source of much human law. Its main limitation is the lack of universal agreement about what behavior is "right," "fair," "just," and "ethical." The affirmative action programs in hiring and medical school admissions for women and minorities in the late 1970s illustrate this problem. By behaving in a manner that probably would be viewed as "fair" by one segment of the population (i.e., giving women and minorities preferential treatment in hiring and medical school admission), one would be behaving in a manner that probably would be viewed as "unfair" by another segment of the population—those who lose jobs and medical school placements to women or minority group members they regard as less qualified than themselves.

Much of our functioning as speech-language pathologists and audiologists is motivated by a desire to do what is *fair*. We believe that our services should be available to any communicatively handicapped person who is likely to profit from them and that it would be *unfair* for such a person to be deprived of them because of an inability to pay. We feel it only *fair* in such instances that a government agency or some other third party pay for the required services. (Such reasoning, incidentally, served as a catalyst for legislation such as P.L. 94-142, which mandated school districts to supply the services required for meeting the special educational needs of all handicapped children in their domains.) We also feel it is *unfair* to keep a person in therapy beyond the point where he or she is likely to profit from it, particularly if the person or the person's family is paying directly for our services.

"Custom Determines Law's Content"

This philosophy suggests that our interpersonal relationships are regulated, in part, by custom or tradition. What has been regarded as acceptable (lawful) behavior is likely to continue to be regarded as such and vice versa. From this perspective, to answer the question "Is X lawful?" we would attempt to determine whether X was viewed as lawful in the past. Court decisions may be made on this basis—that is, on the basis of *precedent*. When handing down a decision a judge usually attempts to justify it, in part, on the basis of how other courts have decided similar cases. (The tendency of judges to base their decisions on precedent, when precedent exists, and thus to not decide what already has been decided is referred to in the legal literature as application of the doctrine of *stare decisis*.) An employer may expect a clinician to function in a certain manner (e.g., maintain a caseload of a particular size or schedule his or her clients in a particular way) because it has been the custom at that institution for clinicians to do so. What is required by custom can be either "good" or "bad," "fair" or "unfair."

Rules (laws) that are not consistent with tradition are likely to be disobeyed.

A classic example of this phenomenon was public reaction to the Eighteenth Amendment to the United States Constitution which prohibited the manufacture and sale of intoxicating liquors for human consumption. This law was unenforceable and had to be repealed by the Twenty-first Amendment.

Clinicians who are prohibited from treating clients they have traditionally been allowed to treat may continue to treat them. School clinicians in one state were told by their department of public instruction to exclude from their caseloads children who had communicative disorders that were not "educationally significant." Nevertheless they frequently found a way to include some of them in their caseloads.

"The Law Is What Legally Constituted Lawmakers Say It Is"

The philosophies that we have discussed—the will of the stronger, the concept of fairness and accepted custom—are not what most persons regard as the content of law. Most people view our legal system as consisting of *rules* (e.g., constitutions, statutes, ordinances, case law made by judges, and administrative regulations) that are promulgated by an individual or a group (e.g., a legislature, court, administrative agency, professional organization, or employer) who are (1) legally authorized to promulgate such rules and (2) have made them in the manner indicated in a constitution (or other document setting forth rule-making procedures) that members of the group have accepted as binding on them. The act of accepting membership in a group, whether citizenship in a country, membership in an organization, or employment in an institution, implies a willingness to accept both the rules and rule-making procedures of that group. Of course, one is free to attempt to change a rule, but one is obligated to do it by means of the procedures outlined in the group's constitution (or other document that specifies rule-changing procedures). This view of law, which is referred to as *positive law,* or *analytical positivism,* is the *main* philosophical foundation of the United States legal system. (The word *main* is used here because all of the philosophies that have been discussed and will be discussed have had impacts on our legal system.)

Rules (laws) promulgated by a group (e.g., the State of Wisconsin, the United States Government, and the American Speech-Language-Hearing Association) who accept this philosophy as the foundation of their legal system have to be accepted by the members of the group *regardless of whether these rules are viewed by them as fair or unfair, desirable or undesirable, and consistent with tradition or not consistent with tradition.* So long as they were made in the appropriate manner and are being promulgated by the appropriate person or persons, the members of the group are expected to obey them. Violation of such a rule is ordinarily supposed to result in sanctions. Possible sanctions include a fine, a jail sentence, or expulsion from the group. Speech-language pathologists and audiologists who are found to be functioning clinically in a manner not consistent with the Code of Ethics of the American Speech-Language-Hearing Association (and thus violating one of its rules) can be expelled from the organization. This would be true even if they viewed the aspect of the Code of Ethics they violated as being unfair or undesirable. During the 1950s and 1960s a number of audiologists were expelled from the association because they violated a part of the code that prohibited their involvement in the dispensing of hearing aids. Some of these audiologists did not obey this part of the code because they viewed it as being unfair or undesirable. (The code was changed during the 1970s to make it possible for audiologists to dispense hearing aids under certain circumstances.) The Ethical Practices Committee was correct in expecting them to obey that part of the code because it was a rule (law) of their association at that time.

"Promote the Greatest Good for the Greatest Number"

This philosophy, which is known as *utilitarianism,* suggests that legislatures (and other law makers) should attempt to promote the greatest good for the greatest number of persons by making appropriate laws (regulations). The desire to promote the greatest good for the greatest number of citizens of the United States undoubtedly motivated such legislation as P.L. 94-142, which mandates school districts to meet the special educational needs of all children in their domains. By promoting the good for a segment of the population, such legislation can be viewed as increasing the good for the entire population. This philosophy also provides a rationale for lobbying for legislation intended to improve the delivery of services to the communicatively handicapped. In addition, the tendency for groups to base decisions on a majority vote also can be viewed as an implicit recognition of this philosophy. The position receiving the most votes usually is the one regarded by those voting as promoting the greatest good for the majority of members of the group. The main limitation of this philosophy is that it can be used to justify ignoring the rights of minorities.

"Conduct Determines the Law"

This philosophy suggests that conduct and law can be interrelated in such a manner that the former will influence the latter. How people behave when confronted by a specific set of circumstances can determine what the law says about how people should behave when confronted by that set of circumstances. The probability that a law will be obeyed is partially a function of how consistent it is with conduct *at the time attempts are made to enforce it.* If a law is significantly at variance with popular conduct—even if it is consistent with custom or tradition—and if the persons who are behaving at variance with the law cannot be convinced of the need to change their behavior, the law is unlikely to be obeyed. Legal penalties associated with the use of marijuana illustrate what can happen if a law is consistent with tradition but not with popular conduct. There were once fairly stringent legal penalties for the possession and use of marijuana, penalties that were consistent with our society's traditional view that the use of marijuana is bad. However, as millions of people representing various segments of the population in the United States began using it, the legal penalties for its possession and use were reduced.

Another example concerns the dispensing of hearing aids by audiologists. Prior to the 1970s audiologists in most professional settings were prohibited from dispensing hearing aids by the Code of Ethics of the American Speech-Language-Hearing Association. Some audiologists, however, felt that dispensing hearing aids was a legitimate aspect of their professional role and did so even though it meant that they could not belong to the association. The Code of Ethics has since been modified to permit audiologists to engage in this activity, thus reconciling law and conduct.

"What the Courts Will Do with Respect to a Particular Matter Is the Law"

This philosophy, known as *functionalism,* suggests that the decision the courts are most likely to make in a particular situation can be regarded as the law in that situation. The emphasis here is on judge-made, or common, law. From this perspective, a court decision must be made on a specific legal problem before one can know what the law is. One implication of this philosophy is that a person can do something that is not prohibited by any legislation or regulations, and that action can be regarded as unlawful at some future date if a court is asked to rule on it. Unfortunately, we are frequently confronted by matters for which the law is unclear and will only become clear when the courts have handed down a decision. The best we can do when confronted by such a situation is to try to predict what the courts will do. Consultation with a lawyer is usually necessary to make such a prediction knowledgeably. The lawyer would attempt to determine through legal research how the courts have decided in somewhat similar situations. Of course, it would be unrealistic to expect any lawyer to be able to predict future rulings with 100 percent accuracy. Thus, the risk of breaking the law can only be minimized, not eliminated.

Uncertainty about what the law is can arise when federal legislation is developed to regulate an area formerly regulated by state legislation. If aspects of the existing state statutes differ from the federal one, which should be obeyed? It could be argued that the federal one should be obeyed because it is *stronger* than (i.e., has precedence over) the state one. It might also be possible to argue that the federal law merely sets *minimum* standards and that the state law because it sets *tougher* standards, should be the applicable one. In such a situation the courts would have to decide what is the law. The potential for this type of court decision existed in some states when the federal law P.L. 94-142 was implemented. Aspects of this law differed from those of some existing state statutes regulating the education of the handicapped. It would have to be left to the courts to decide what is the law on these aspects.

"Unconscious Prejudices Influence Court Decisions"

The philosophies considered thus far have dealt with the law as if its interpretation were independent of the person or persons interpreting it. They implicitly assume that the motivations and prejudices of lawmakers and interpreters (e.g., judges and juries) do not influence the content of law and how it is interpreted and applied. In other words, they seem to assume that "justice is blind." Such an assumption is counterintuitive. There is a philosophy known as *realism* that does take such factors into consideration when defining law. Those who accept this philosophy view the law *as we know it* as involving an interaction between the observer and the observed (Johnson, 1946). The observers' (e.g., judges or juries) attitudes are regarded as influencing how they interpret the observed (the law). Fisher has noted:

> In deciding cases it was perceived that unconscious prejudices judges held respecting the likelihood of someone's having committed a crime, the judge's view of the good or evil that motivated a defendant, and the basic likes and dislikes of the judge, affect a decision more than applicable rules. Realists believed superficialities such as dress, skin color, age, occupation, and vocabulary were unacknowledged factors entering into the calculus determinative of criminal guilt or innocence or civil liability or nonliability. Juries' prejudices similarly influence their verdicts quite apart from objective evidence. (Fisher, 1977, p. 19)

Such extraneous factors, of course, enter into the administration (enforcement) of rules at all levels. A given infraction is apt to be reacted to, in part, on the basis of the perceived status of the person breaking the rule. The higher the rule breaker's perceived status, the weaker the penalty is apt to be. An administrator who breaks a rule (e.g., arrives at work late) is apt to be dealt with less severely by an employer than an unskilled worker who breaks the same rule.

How can the impact of such factors be reduced? Perhaps this can be accomplished, in part, by heightening the awareness of those administering law about the manner in which their unconscious prejudices can influence their decision making. At any rate, we should constantly be aware that decision makers can be influenced by such factors and, if possible, use such factors to our advantage rather than disadvantage. If we are asked to appear in court as expert witnesses, we should attempt to create the kind of image that will communicate high credibility.

"Law Inhibits or Frustrates Our Instincts"

We have viewed law thus far from the prospective of its impact on the overt behavior of those who are subjected to it. We have considered how laws can influence interpersonal relationships by imposing restrictions and obligations on our functioning in such relationships. Law also can be viewed from the perspective of its impacts on our *covert*, or internal physiological, functioning. It can influence our emotional status by frustrating our instincts. (One of the first persons, incidentally, to point this out was Sigmund Freud, the founder of psychoanalysis.) How can law-related frustration affect our emotional functioning?

> There are obvious individual costs of law's being a frustration mechanism: ulcers, high blood pressure, heart attacks, neuroses, and other psychological

(7) On June 22, 1971, the dean expelled Robert from Hofstra, severing him from the University "completely and permanently." He barred Robert from any part of the campus without his express prior permission under pain of arrest as a trespasser. Finally, he fined Robert and his family $1,011.61 for the ostensible cost of replacing the windows.

(8) At no time prior to his expulsion, barring and fining, was Robert given a choice of procedure, was he represented by any counsel, nor did he have an opportunity to confront any witnesses, nor was he interviewed by any school psychologist or medical personnel.

(9) The dean claims that Robert was guilty of the rock-throwing charges, and that in light of these and the other uncharged incidents he was troublesome and emotionally disturbed. Robert claims he is innocent, that his confession was pressured from him, and that the university is and has been harassing him because of his tuition protest activities.

(10) The Hofstra Disciplinary Regulations for Nonacademic Conduct provide that when the dean of students is advised of an incident possibly requiring disciplinary action he may either interview the student himself or refer the matter to a member of his staff. Upon determining that disciplinary hearing is appropriate, the student is given a choice of appearing before either a student judiciary board or members of the dean of student's staff.

(11) The dean specified in his testimony that Robert was not given a choice of the student judiciary board, based on that portion of the Hofstra rules which provide that a student "whose records suggest significant emotional or psychological disturbances which may be relevant" will be heard only by the dean's staff. The dean did not consult any psychologist or psychiatrist before making the disciplinary reference to his staff committee. The testimony was that the staff committee concerned itself with emotional disturbance upon talking with a university psychologist.

(12) There are no rules as to the procedures of the dean's staff committee except that its members present their recommendations to the dean. The dean must then interview the student and give his decision. Hofstra's rules do provide an "appeal" procedure for non-academic disciplinary situations. If the student believes that the dean's punishment is inappropriate, he may have a hearing by a review committee of five university staff and faculty members and two students upon his petition submitted to the vice president for student affairs within ten days after penalty. The vice president is then supposed to advise the student of his right to call witnesses on his behalf and to confront and cross-examine those who appear against him and of his right to seek counsel, which counsel is limited, however, only to a university staff or faculty member.

(13) The review committee is charged with examining the evidence, hearing witnesses as to the facts and the student's character, and weighing extenuating circumstances. The administration, but not the student, has a further right of appeal to the university board of trustees.

(14) During June, Robert orally requested of the dean and the Hofstra vice president of student affairs a hearing, but was told that he had to petition in writing. A lawyer representing Robert requested an appeal hearing by letter dated July 9, 1971, to the dean. This letter was returned to the lawyer suggesting that the request be directed to the university vice president for student affairs. Thereupon, the attorney mailed a similar letter to that official on July 23, 1971, requesting that the review be held prior to the fall semester, but the administration took no action on this.

(15) On August 4, 1971, Robert requested that because of family illness the hearing be delayed until the fall and that he be permitted to attend classes pending the completion of the appeal. This request was turned down by the vice president for student affairs on August 9, 1971, who volunteered that Robert's right to petition for a hearing was extended to September 1, 1971. On August 26, 1971, Robert wrote personally to the vice president for student affairs requesting an appeal. On September 9, 1971, Robert received a letter (dated September 1st) from an assistant president stating that there was no more vice president for student affairs, advising Robert that he would be notified of a hearing date "as soon as practicable," and directing communication to him.

(16) On September 14, 1971, without any further word from the administration as to review, Robert commenced this proceeding to compel Hofstra to readmit him to classes. On September 16, 1971, classes reopened at Hofstra for the fall season. Sometime after the hearing of this judicial proceeding on September 23, 1971, a review proceeding was first scheduled for October 5, 1971.

(17) Essentially, Robert's contention is that the university's action was improper and arbitrary and that the proceedings deprived him of due process of law. In reply, Hofstra asserts that the university acted properly and that Hofstra, as a private institution, was not legally obliged to afford fair process to its students. Hofstra argues that since it is a private university it suffers no restriction at all in its disciplining of its students. However one gauges the contemporaneous sensitivity of this attitude, it is plainly not the law. Whatever the application to this case, there are some limits.

(18) The dean testified that he gave Robert no choice of appearing before the student judiciary board because of that provision of the rules requiring staff referral only for "students whose records suggest significant emotional or psychological disturbance." Even though Robert was sent to the staff committee and given no student judiciary board choice because of an assumed record of emotional or psychological disturbance, Robert was at no time interviewed by any medical or psychological personnel, nor were any records produced suggesting the offending disturbance.

(19) Under the adopted rules, Robert was entitled to a student judiciary board choice unless the record suggested significant emotional disturbance on his part. There was no proof of any such record prior to his referral to the dean's committee. It was indeed the reverse. It was the staff committee which raised the emotional concern after the student judiciary board choice had already been withheld.

(20) Accordingly, in the absence of a foundation for his conduct, the dean acted arbitrarily and in abuse of discretion in not giving Robert the choice of appearing before a student judiciary board as required by the Hofstra rules.

(21) Implicit in the rules must be a requirement for the university to act with reasonable promptness on review applications. The testimony reflects without doubt that the Hofstra administration delayed materially in scheduling a review hearing. Where after oral notification, it had a written notice on July 9, 1971, and subsequent written requests on July 23rd and August 26th, it first scheduled an appeal hearing on October 5, 1971, three weeks after school reopened. And this scheduling came only after the court hearing in this proceeding.

(22) Given the time necessary to conduct an appeal and reach a reasoned decision, it is apparent that the procedure adopted will necessarily deprive Robert of a semester's attendance in class, or at best put him under an onerous make-up schedule, if possible, even if he is totally successful on appeal.

(23) This delay works the imposition of a significant penalty which entirely bypasses the review procedure, and must be termed arbitrary and capricious, and abusive of discretion, on the part of the Hofstra administration.

(24) The university's insistence on a written petition in Robert's personal hand to the vice president for student affairs as an excuse for delay is hypertechnical and not legitimate justification. After oral notice from Robert, it rejected the first written communication from his lawyer because it was addressed to the moving and visible dean and not to a certain vice president, and then rejected the lawyer's written request to the officer to which it directed him on the ground that Robert personally, not a lawyer, had to write out the request. The administration was fully and fairly informed by the lawyer's letters of July 9, 1971, to the dean of students and of July 23, 1971, to the vice president of student affairs. A lawyer acts as a personal representative of his client and for him. The administration's treatment of this simple request for review smacks of a "runaround." Moreover, if technicality is the order of the day, nothing in the rules precludes petition by a lawyer writing on behalf of a student, unlike the review procedures which specifically limit right to counsel. Amusingly enough, even the administration departed from its insistence on communications with one indispensable officer as the touchstone for its procedure, for in August Hofstra dispensed with its position of vice president for student affairs altogether. After Robert had personally petitioned that requisite officer, it turned out the office no longer existed, and the university itself requested Robert to communicate with some assistant president. Even then it delayed for six more weeks until October 5, 1971.

(25) Finally, the hasty imposition on Robert and his family of a money fine in excess of $1000 for three separate incidents, of which only one had a claimed eyewitness, without even submitted proof of damage, was precipitous. The family was not heard at all and in no way signed for any responsibility. A particularly unreasonable part of the skimpy procedure here is that the expelled student cannot get a transcript to enable transfer admission to another school until he pays the fine to the university. Accordingly, a student is put into the position of being required to pay or prosecute a successful appeal, no matter the time delay, before he can transfer to another school. This financial obligation springs into existence without benefit of counsel or fair hearing.

(26) In Dixon v. Alabama Board of Education, 294 F.2d 150, the court held a student could not be expelled from a tax supported university without notice and some opportunity to be heard. In defining "due process," the court emphasized that the nature of the hearing depended on the circum-

stances of the particular case. It said that "full dress judicial hearings" are not required, because they are not appropriate to college context, but that the requirements of due process are fulfilled by having "the rudimentary elements of fair play." There must be "every semblance of fairness" in school disciplinary procedure. Due process is then a variable thing. Something different is called for by a criminal trial than a college disciplinary proceeding. But, the constant factor is that the procedure afforded must be traditionally fair and conscionable in the context taken.

(27) Bearing in mind that this is a college disciplinary matter, and not a criminal trial (although the acts charged are crimes and admissions taken damaging), it must be observed that Robert's treatment fell short of the rudimentary requirements of fair play.

(28) In the collegiate context, the initial nonacademic discipline procedure at Hofstra is not unreasonable, provided it is followed. Since the subsequent appeal or review procedure contemplates an open hearing with witnesses and confrontation, the juxtaposition is not inconsistent with the need to keep order. But when the prescribed procedure is not followed, when punitive delay is set in, and when excessive punishment is summarily dealt, the administration violates the necessary rudiments of fair play.

(29) Based on the findings and principles set forth above, the action of the Hofstra University dean in expelling Robert Ryan, Jr., barring him from the campus, and fining him and his family will be nullified.

This court opinion is representative of the types of information that usually are included and the manner in which they are organized. If you were to look up the decision made in a case in which you were interested at a law library, it probably would be structured similarly. We have indexed the headings and paragraphs with letters and numbers to facilitate our discussion.

The first line of the heading (line *a*) presents the *case name*. The *plaintiff* (the person or institution who is suing) ordinarily is mentioned first and the *defendant* (the person or institution being sued) second. Line *b* is the *bibliographical reference* to the volume in which the opinion was printed. Line *c* gives the *name of the court* in which the judge handing down the decision presides, and line *d* indicates the *date the opinion was released*. The *name of the judge* who wrote the opinion is indicated at the beginning of the first paragraph.

A court opinion, according to Rombauer, ideally should contain *five* well-defined parts. The first of these is "a statement of the significant facts of the dispute before the court—the facts that are necessary for an understanding of the dispute and of the court's decision, those that influenced the court's reasoning and decision" (1978, p. 8). This information is presented in paragraphs three through nine of Judge Harnett's opinion.

A second type of information that Rombauer states should be included in an opinion is "a statement of the relevant procedural details. This would include an explanation of the legal nature of the controversy and of the remedy sought . . . and of the relevant procedural actions taken in the lower court" (1978, p. 8). The remedy sought here by Robert is having his being barred from the university and his fine nullified. Relevant information on procedural details is presented in paragraphs 10 through 18.

A third type of information that Rombauer indicates should be included in an opinion is "a statement of the narrow legal question(s) or issue(s) that the ... court was asked to resolve" (1978, p. 8). This question here is whether Hofstra, as a *private* institution, is *legally obliged* to adhere to a particular set of procedures when disciplining its students (i.e., procedures that would be consistent with the doctrine of *due process of law*). This question is implied by the discussion in paragraphs 1 and 17.

A fourth type of information that Rombauer indicates should be included in an opinion is "a brief statement of the ... court's decision, both procedural (e.g., judgment for plaintiff is affirmed) and substantive (a "yes" or "no" answer for each question)" (1978, p. 8). That for the *procedural* aspect is presented in paragraph 29 of the opinion and that for the *substantive* aspect is presented in the last two sentences of paragraph 17.

The final type of information that Rombauer indicates should be included in an opinion is "an explanation of the court's reasoning in reaching its decision. This explanation might include what is sometimes treated as a sixth important part of an opinion: a statement of a general principle or rule assumed or found to preexist from which the court reasoned or a statement of the narrow rule that the court applied or developed in reaching its decision" (1978, p. 8). The explanation for the decision reached in this case is summarized in paragraphs 18 through 28.

The opinion that is reproduced here was selected because it is both clearly written (i.e., it contains very little legal jargon) and illustrates well the various parts of a typical opinion. Since it was issued by a lower (trial) court rather than a court of appeals or a state or federal supreme court, it probably would have very little impact as a molder of legal precedent.

The process through which court opinions are transformed into law by application of the doctrine of *stare decisis* can be summarized as follows:

> Given a determination of the facts in a dispute, *assuming no controlling law* [italics added], a court decides the case on the basis of what it believes the law is or should be. In determining what the law is or should be, it looks first to prior decisions resolving similar or analogous disputes and seeks to apply the underlying rules or principles that appear to have been established by those decisions. If the facts presented to the court include the same significant facts as appeared in a previously decided case, without additional facts that could be regarded as significant, the court frequently will bow to the authority of the decision in the prior case and follow it, reaching the same result in the pending case.... If no prior decided case presented the same significant facts, the court will consider whether any prior decided case nevertheless has sufficient elements in common with the pending dispute to require or justify application of a rule or principle derivable from or underlying the decision in such prior case. (Rombauer, 1978, p. 5)

The phrase "assuming no controlling written law" was italicized to highlight the fact that if there is a controlling written law that applies to the facts in a case, the

ject matter (e.g., juveniles). Others have *general jurisdiction:* They are authorized to handle any subject matter.
4. Does the suit involve a question of violation of a federal statute (or statutes)? Examples would be cases claiming violations in the area of civil rights or of copyrights. Federal courts usually have jurisdiction in such cases, regardless of the amount of money involved.
5. Which court, of those that will accept jurisdiction, is most likely to decide in favor of the client? The attorney for the plaintiff may find, based on a court's (or judge's) record of decisions in similar cases that it may or may not be advantageous for the case to be tried in that court (or by that judge). Given a choice, lawyers will select that court (or judge) most likely to decide for their clients.

The court (or judge) selected by the plaintiff in a civil action will not usually be changed unless the defendant can show that there are very good reasons for doing so.

Legislatures

The most readily apparent sources from which laws originate are municipal (city), state, and federal legislatures. A legislature is "a body of public officials who collectively have the authority to make generalized law for future application" (Grilliot, 1979, p. 550). Those who serve as members of legislatures in almost all instances are elected to serve in this capacity for a specified period of time by geographically defined groups of people *whose interests they are supposed to represent.* Such a geographically defined group (or *constituency)* could consist of persons who live in a particular section of a large city or in one of several adjacent smaller cities. Presumably, a legislator's constituents can motivate him or her to represent their interests by indicating through face-to-face contact, a telephone call, a letter, or a telegram that they intend to exercise their right to vote when he or she runs for reelection. Even a relatively small number of letters or telegrams from constituents indicating why they believe their legislators should vote in a particular way on a particular bill can significantly affect the outcome of the vote on that bill. (This topic is dealt with further in Chapter 12, on lobbying.) The legislative branch of a municipal (local) government is variously referred to by such terms as the city council, the board of aldermen, or the common council. The legislative branch of state government is referred to as the state legislature and that of the federal government as the United States Congress.

Both state and federal legislatures consist of two branches, with the exception of Nebraska, which has a unicameral legislature. The more prestigious of the two, known as the Senate, usually has fewer members than the other, which is known as the House of Representatives or State Assembly. Thus, senators tend to represent a larger constituency than do members of the House of Representatives.

The authority for Congress to exercise its lawmaking function is contained in Article 1 of the United States Constitution (see Appendix D). In Section 18 of this article it states that Congress shall have the power "To make all laws which shall be necessary and proper for carrying into Execution ... all ... powers vested by this Constitution in the Government of the United States, or any department or office thereof." The Constitution thus gives Congress broad authority for making laws. It also places limits on this lawmaking ability. The framers (and amenders) of the Constitution prohibited Congress from making certain types of laws to protect what they regarded as inalienable rights of United States citizens. Included here are *ex post facto laws* "which make a crime of an act which when committed was not a crime" (Black, 1968, p. 662). A hypothetical example of the application of an *ex post facto* law would be a speech-language pathologist or audiologist being charged with violating the Code of Ethics of the American Speech-Language-Hearing Association because he or she violated an aspect of this code *that was not a part of it* at the time he or she failed to function in compliance with it. These restrictions on the lawmaking function of Congress also include limitations on the power to pass laws (1) restricting religion, speech, the press, and the right to assemble peaceably (First Amendment) and (2) depriving people of life, liberty, or property without *due process of law* (Fifth Amendment). See Article 1 and the Amendments to the Constitution (Appendix D) for other restrictions on Congress's lawmaking function.

The authority for state legislatures to exercise their lawmaking functions "to preserve the public health, safety, morals, and welfare" (Grilliot, 1979, p. 338) existed prior to the framing of the United States Constitution and hence was not derived from it. The legislatures of the thirteen colonies had assumed this function because of their belief in the right of every *sovereignty* (i.e., governmental unit) to pass laws for its internal regulation. This right was accepted without reservation by the framers of the Constitution, although they did set limits on the types of subject matter about which state legislatures could pass laws (see Article 1, Section 10, of the Constitution, included in Appendix D). The Tenth Amendment states that "The powers not delegated to the United States by the Constitution, nor prohibited by it to the States, are reserved to the States respectively, or to the people." Municipal governmental units derive authority for their lawmaking functions on a similar basis—that is, the right of a governmental unit to pass laws for its internal regulation within limits set by state and federal constitutions.

The process by which proposed laws *(bills)* are transformed by a legislature (federal, state, or municipal) into laws *(statutes)* consists of an ordered series of steps that are specified in the constitution of the sovereignty. For the U.S. Congress, these steps are specified in Article 1, Sections 5 and 7 of the Constitution. Article 7 delineates the broad outlines of this process. Article 5, by giving the House of Representatives and Senate authority to "determine the rules of its proceedings," mandates the development of a set of procedures that would result in the Congress's functioning as indicated in Article 7. For a particular state or municipal legislature, at least the broad outlines of these steps would be suggested in the constitution of that state or municipality.

The steps (or decision points) that a bill must survive before becoming a statute are ordered. This ordering for a typical bill proposed in the U.S. Congress is indicated in Figure 2-5. A detailed description of the process by which legislatures

This graphic shows the most typical way in which proposed legislation is enacted into law. There are more complicated, as well as simpler, routes, and most bills fall by the wayside and never become law. The process is illustrated with two hypothetical bills, House bill No. 1 (HR 1) and Senate bill No. 2 (S 2). Each bill must be passed by both houses of Congress in identical form before it can become law. The path of HR 1 is traced by a solid line, that of S 2 by a broken line. However, in practice most legislation begins as similar proposals in both houses.

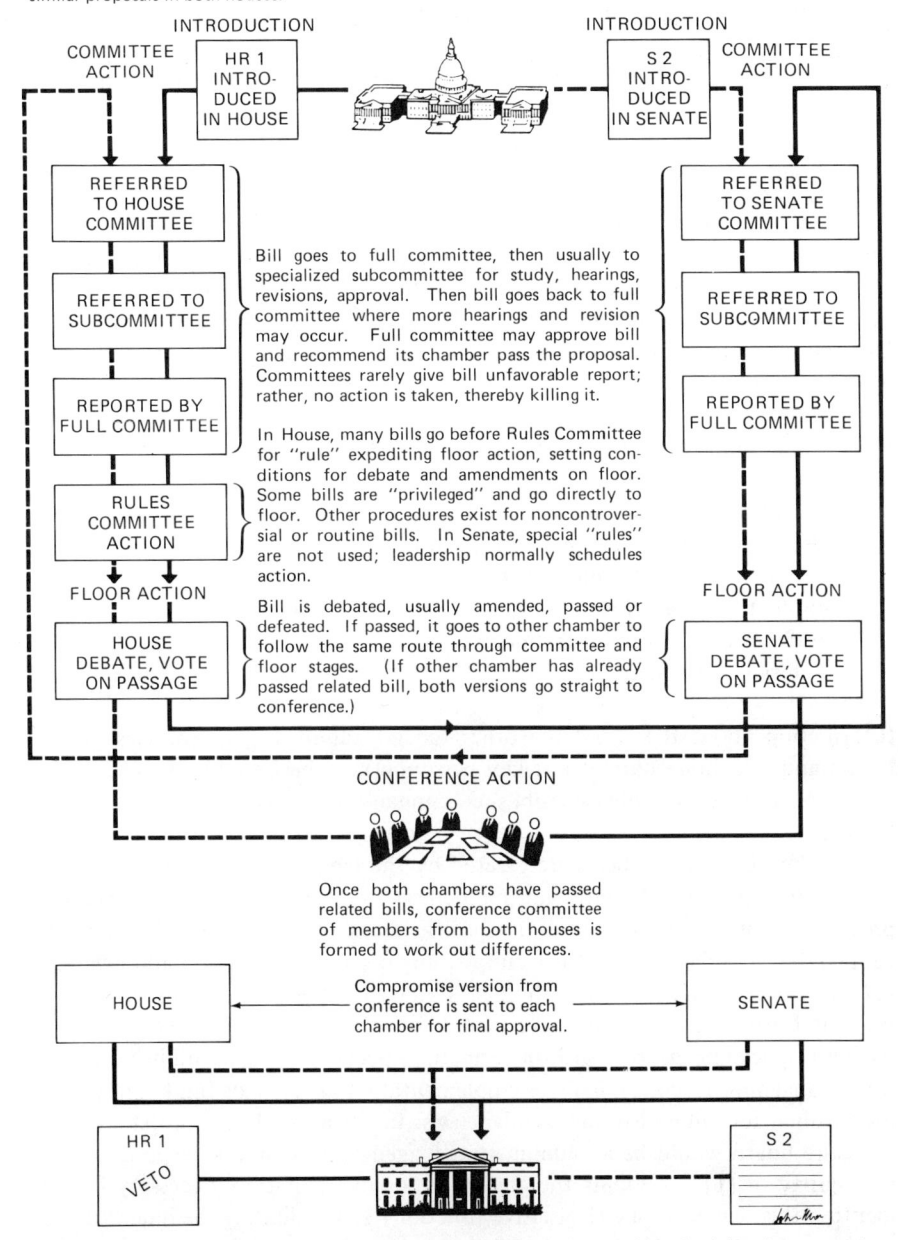

INTRODUCTION

COMMITTEE ACTION

HR 1 INTRODUCED IN HOUSE

REFERRED TO HOUSE COMMITTEE

REFERRED TO SUBCOMMITTEE

REPORTED BY FULL COMMITTEE

RULES COMMITTEE ACTION

FLOOR ACTION

HOUSE DEBATE, VOTE ON PASSAGE

Bill goes to full committee, then usually to specialized subcommittee for study, hearings, revisions, approval. Then bill goes back to full committee where more hearings and revision may occur. Full committee may approve bill and recommend its chamber pass the proposal. Committees rarely give bill unfavorable report; rather, no action is taken, thereby killing it.

In House, many bills go before Rules Committee for "rule" expediting floor action, setting conditions for debate and amendments on floor. Some bills are "privileged" and go directly to floor. Other procedures exist for noncontroversial or routine bills. In Senate, special "rules" are not used; leadership normally schedules action.

Bill is debated, usually amended, passed or defeated. If passed, it goes to other chamber to follow the same route through committee and floor stages. (If other chamber has already passed related bill, both versions go straight to conference.)

INTRODUCTION

COMMITTEE ACTION

S 2 INTRODUCED IN SENATE

REFERRED TO SENATE COMMITTEE

REFERRED TO SUBCOMMITTEE

REPORTED BY FULL COMMITTEE

FLOOR ACTION

SENATE DEBATE, VOTE ON PASSAGE

CONFERENCE ACTION

Once both chambers have passed related bills, conference committee of members from both houses is formed to work out differences.

HOUSE ← Compromise version from conference is sent to each chamber for final approval. → SENATE

HR 1 VETO

S 2

Compromise version approved by both houses is sent to President who can either sign it into law or veto it and return it to Congress. Congress may override veto by a two-thirds majority vote in both houses; bill then becomes law without President's signature.

FIGURE 2-5 How a bill becomes law. (Adapted from GUIDE TO CONGRESS, Second Edition. Washington, D.C.: Congressional Quarterly, Inc., 1976.)

create law is being presented here because an intuitive understanding of this process is a prerequisite for influencing it. Speech-language pathologists and audiologists should obviously be interested in influencing legislation that affects both their professional functioning (e.g., third-party payments for their services under federal insurance programs) and the providing of services to the communicatively handicapped.

Administrative Agencies

Administrative agencies are rule-making (lawmaking) organizations that exist in all federal, state, and municipal governments. They may be referred to as commissions, services, boards, authorities, bureaus, offices, departments, corporations, administrations, divisions, or agencies. Those in the federal government that regulate the activities of speech-language pathologists and audiologists include the following:

Equal Employment Opportunity Commission
Internal Revenue Service
Occupational Safety and Health Review Commission
Department of Education (Special Education Programs)
Office of Human Development
Public Health Service
Social Security Administration
Veterans Administration

Information about these and the other federal administrative agencies (including names and telephone numbers of key personnel) can be found in the *United States Government Manual,* which is published annually by the U.S. Government Printing Office.

Administrative agencies are created by the legislative and executive branches of government (federal, state, and municipal) to develop, administer, and enforce programs they have mandated in specific areas (e.g., education of the handicapped). A state legislature, for example, might pass a bill that would regulate the activities of speech-language pathologists and audiologists by licensure. To implement it the legislature would have included in the bill provisions either for establishing a special licensure board for regulating speech, language, and hearing services or for assigning responsibility for implementation to an existing board (e.g., one responsible for administering similar laws for health-related professions). This licensure board would be an administrative agency. It would be responsible for the nitty-gritty of (1) developing the guidelines, or rules, that are necessary for implementing this licensure law (legislative function); (2) evaluating the qualifications of persons who wish to be licensed under it and, if their qualifications are adequate, granting them licenses (executive function); and (3) policing persons who have been licensed and if necessary conducting hearings that could result in suspension or revocation of their licenses (judicial function). Almost all administrative agencies, as we have indicated in this example, perform executive, legislative, and judicial functions. Thus, they do not appear to adhere to the concept of separation of powers that, judging by the Constitution, is a fundamental aspect of our form of government. (This aspect of their functioning has been challenged on constitutional grounds, but apparently not successfully.)

Administrative agencies are not mentioned directly in the Constitution. They owe their existence to the legislative and executive branches of government. Congress, theoretically, can terminate any federal administrative agency by merely passing a statute. Adminstrative agencies were originally established to implement legislation at relatively low cost with as few mistakes as possible. It was believed that it would be more costly to have the members of Congress develop the rules for implementing a statute than to have a group of relatively low-paid bureaucrats do so. Moreover, a group of bureaucrats with expertise in the specific subject matter area of the legislation would probably be less likely to make errors as they established rules than would members of Congress, most of whom probably would lack expertise in the subject matter. Of course, concluding that administrative agencies, because of their expertise, would be less likely to make errors in rule making than would the Congress is not the same as concluding that they do not make errors. No decision-making process involving humans can be error-free. Rules that are either unreasonable or undesirable (or both) are promulgated by administrative agencies. However, when rules adopted by administrative agencies are viewed as unreasonable or undesirable, they can be challenged in the courts. Also, administrative agencies can be ordered to eliminate some of their rules if an administration wishes to reduce regulation, or deregulate.

The procedure that an administrative agency follows for rule making is supposed to permit input from anyone. Those that *federal* administrative agencies are required to follow, which are summarized here, illustrate how such input can influence this process.

> The basic procedural idea is quite simple: An agency prepares a proposed rule after whatever study and investigation and consultation it finds desirable, publishes it, invites written comments on it, reworks it in the light of the comments, and then issues the final rule. Sometimes the agency hears oral arguments. Sometimes it issues a second proposed rule. Sometimes, when issues of specific fact call for such procedure, the agency conducts a trial-type hearing on those issues. The procedure is flexible and the variations depend upon circumstances and special needs.
> Much experience shows that the procedure is efficient, fair, democratic, and easy. A small party may write a letter to point out how a proposed rule will affect him, to request a slight alteration, and to make an argument. A big company may make an elaborate study, present the detailed results, and ask for opportunity for its lawyers to present oral argument. The agency will summarize the main new facts and ideas and explain the reasons for the

choices it makes. Anyone has the opportunity to propose changes not only in proposed rules but even in rules that have been adopted. (Davis, 1977, p. 241)

The procedure that would be used by state and municipal administrative agencies for obtaining public input on proposed rules would be quite similar in most instances.

How can one keep informed about new rules being proposed by administrative agencies? For federal administrative agencies, most (but not all) of these are published in a periodical distributed by the U.S. Government Printing Office known as the *Federal Register.* It also includes information about new rules that have been adopted by these agencies. Most states and municipalities, unfortunately, do not have a publication comparable to the *Federal Register.* Although it is almost always possible to obtain information about new rules being proposed by state and municipal administrative agencies, the information usually cannot be obtained as conveniently as for the federal agencies.

Rules, guidelines, and other records generated by federal agencies that are not published in the *Federal Register* can often be obtained directly from these agencies by requesting the information under the terms of the *Freedom of Information Act.* The word *often* is italicized because (1) this act requires the person requesting a document to *specifically identify* it and (2) the act contains a list of exemptions; if an agency can show that the information requested is covered by one or more of these exemptions, it can refuse to release the information.

Why might a speech-language pathologist or audiologist request information from a federal agency under the *Freedom of Information Act?* One reason could be to obtain the full set of reviewers' comments on a grant application they had submitted. If a speech-language pathologist or audiologist is dissatisfied with the information received from an agency about why a grant application was rejected, he or she can request a copy of the file on the application under the terms of this act.

Professional Organizations

Professional organizations, such as the American Speech-Language-Hearing Association, are not usually regarded as possible sources of law because they are not a component of municipal, state, or federal government. Yet they often function in this role, particularly if they certify the professional competence of their members and develop, administer, and enforce a code of ethics. The influence they exert over their members when functioning in this capacity is comparable to that exerted by a municipal, state, or federal *administrative agency* over its constituents. The type of administrative agency that an organization functioning in this way would appear to be most comparable to is a state professional licensing board. In awarding its Certificate of Clinical Competence in Speech Pathology and Certificate of Clinical Competence in Audiology, the American Speech-Language-Hearing Association functions similarly to such a board. (However, it should be noted that ASHA certification is voluntary; state licenses ordinarily are not.) The association performs legislative, executive, and judicial functions: It establishes the requirements for the certificates (legislative function); it evaluates the qualifications of persons who wish to be awarded one or both of the certificates (executive function); and it monitors the activities of persons who have been awarded them (judicial function).

Information about new rules under consideration by professional organizations and recently adopted rules are usually published in one of the organizations' journals. Such information is published by the American Speech-Language-Hearing Association in the journal *Asha.*

HOW ARE THE LAWS THAT MAKE UP OUR LEGAL SYSTEM CATEGORIZED?

Having examined the *sources* from which we get the laws that make up our legal system, we shall now consider the laws themselves and specifically, some of the terms used for categorizing them. An intuitive understanding of the meanings of such terms (categories), of course, can help us understand the intended function of laws within the categories.

All rules (laws) that are intended to influence our behavior, regardless of their origin, can be assigned to one of three *content* categories: criminal, administrative, or civil (see Figure 2-6). *Criminal laws* deal with crimes, or acts against society. Such acts can be against a municipal or state government, the federal government, or the international community (e.g., genocide). Some deviations from society's behavioral expectations, or crimes, are viewed as more serious than are others. Relatively minor ones, such as parking your car in a no-parking zone, are classified as *misdemeanors;* more serious ones are classified as *felonies.* Misdemeanors usually are punishable by relatively low fines and/or relatively short terms of imprisonment. Felonies are punishable by relatively large fines, relatively long terms of imprisonment, and in some extremely serious cases, such as treason, death. One is accused of committing a crime by a representative of the governmental unit against which it was supposedly committed, usually a district attorney. When a criminal

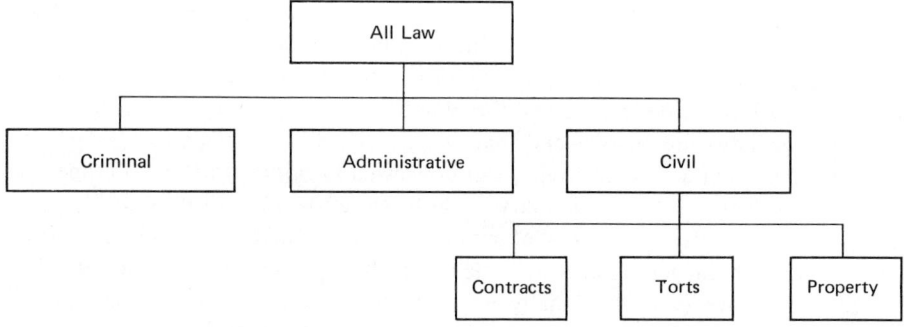

FIGURE 2-6 Some types of law that are professionally relevant.

```
                        All Law
          ┌───────────────┼───────────────┐
       Criminal      Administrative       Civil
                                   ┌────────┼────────┐
                               Contracts  Torts   Property
```

case is tried in a court, it ordinarily is titled *people* versus the name of the defendant (e.g., *People* v. *Silverman*). This convention highlights the fact that what the person is accused of doing is contrary to the interests of society—that is, the people. In such court proceedings the defendant is presumed to be innocent: He or she can be found guilty only if the people can establish guilt *beyond a shadow of a doubt*— for example if the members of a jury conclude the defendant is guilty.

Administrative law deals with regulations promulgated by municipal, state, and federal administrative agencies. Information about such agencies as a source of law is presented in the preceding section of this chapter.

Civil law is concerned with relationships between private individuals (rather than between private individuals and society, which is the concern of criminal law). We all enter into many such relationships, and when doing so we implicitly or explicitly accept restrictions and obligations. Civil law deals with those restrictions and obligations intended to protect the rights of private individuals. It makes them explicit and offers *procedures* for resolving controversies involving them. These procedures include the *civil suit*, in which "the court attempts to remedy the controversy between individuals by determining their legal rights, awarding money damages to the injured party, or directing one party to do or refrain from doing a specific act" (Grilliot, 1979, p. 23).

There are several types (categories) of civil law. Those that are professionally relevant to speech-language pathologists and audiologists include *contracts, torts*, and *property*.

Contract law is intended to facilitate interpersonal relationships. For a society to exist in which individuals are not completely self-sufficient (which would be any society) its members have to *cooperate*. Few individuals can provide for themselves more than a small number of the goods and services they require for their survival. They must rely on others for most of them. The agreement by which these goods and services are provided is known as a *contract*. A contract is "a promise, or set of promises, for *breach* of which the law gives a *remedy*, or the performance of which the law in some way recognizes as a *duty*" (Gifis, 1975, p. 44). The role of contracts in clinical practice is dealt with in Chapter 4.

Torts are injuries or wrongs to individuals resulting from the dangerous or unreasonable conduct of others, *that do not arise from breaching (not fulfilling) a contract*, for which courts will provide a remedy by awarding compensation. The assumption here, of course, is that the injuries or wrongs can be proven to have resulted from dangerous or unreasonable conduct by the defendant. Torts differ from crimes in that crimes are injuries or wrongs to *society*, and torts are injuries or wrongs to *private individuals*. Thus, the plaintiff (accuser) in a court case involving a crime is society—the people—and that in a court case involving a tort is a private individual. A given act, incidentally, can be viewed as *both* a tort and a crime if it can be proven to have caused injury to both society and a private individual (or group of individuals). The types of wrongs or injuries that one person can do to another through dangerous or unreasonable conduct (which are the types of torts) include negligence (a professionally relevant aspect of which is malpractice), invasion of privacy, defamation (as in saying or writing something false about another

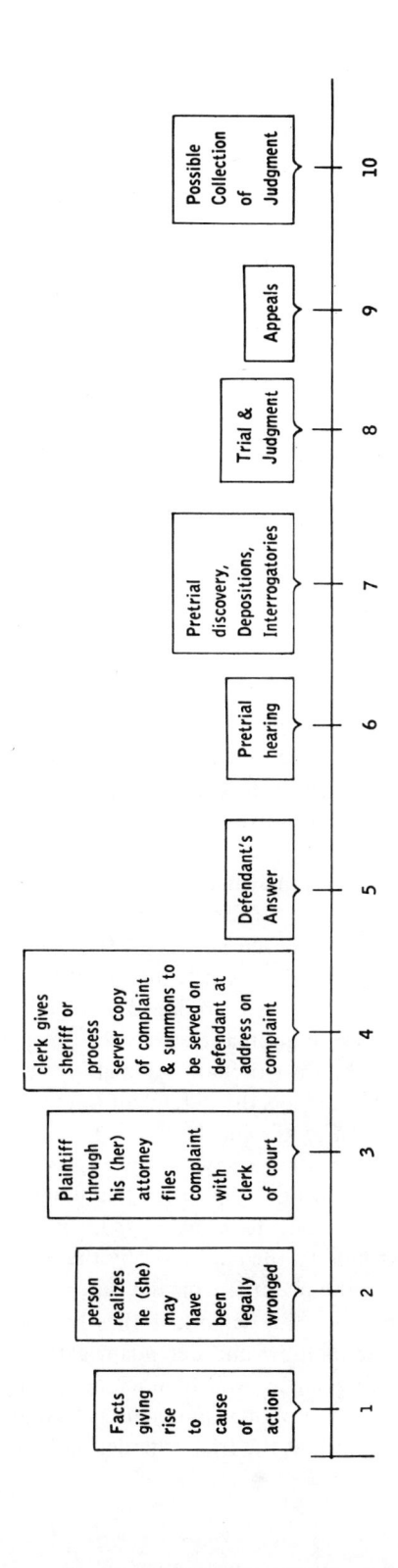

```
1          2          3            4            5          6         7            8          9          10
Facts      person     Plaintiff    clerk gives  Defendant's Pretrial  Pretrial    Trial &    Appeals    Possible
giving     realizes   through      sheriff or   Answer     hearing   discovery,  Judgment              Collection
rise       he (she)   his (her)    process                           Depositions,                      of
to         may        attorney     server copy                       Interrogatories                   Judgment
cause      have been  files        of complaint
of         legally    complaint    & summons to
action     wronged    with clerk   be served on
                      of court     defendant at
                                   address on
                                   complaint
```

FIGURE 2-8 Steps in a civil lawsuit. (Reprinted by permission from INTRODUCTION TO THE LEGAL SYSTEM, Second Edition by Bruce D. Fisher. Copyright © 1977 by West Publishing Company. All rights reserved.)

the *defendant*. If the defendant can convince the court that the plaintiff has waited too long to initiate the suit, he or she can avoid having to be a party to it. The attorney for the defendant may raise the issue of the statute of limitations at the beginning of the lawsuit in an effort to end the suit.

Once a person becomes aware of having been legally wronged and decides to seek a judicial remedy—to initiate a lawsuit—he or she will first contact an attorney (or a law firm) who is willing to present his or her *complaint* to a court. This, of course, assumes that the person decided not to act *pro se* (i.e., as his or her own attorney). If the attorney feels after hearing the complaint and doing some informal investigation that the suit being proposed has merit and the person is likely to be awarded the remedy being sought, the attorney is likely to agree to represent the person on either a fixed fee or contingency fee basis. (Considerations relevant to the choice between them are discussed elsewhere in this chapter.) The attorney will then draft a *written complaint* that indicates why the client (the plaintiff in the suit being initiated) believes he or she was legally wronged by the defendant, and what judicial remedy is being sought. A representative example of such a complaint is reproduced in Figure 2-9. The original and two copies are delivered to the *clerk of the court* in which the plaintiff intends to initiate the suit. The clerk stamps the three copies with the date and time of day, keeps the original, returns one copy to the plaintiff, and gives the second copy to an *official process server* along with a *summons*, which directs the defendant to appear in court to answer the complaint. The process server delivers the copy of the complaint and the summons to the person who will be the defendant in the suit. (In some suits the defendant may be an organization.) This serves as official notification to the defendant that he or she is being sued.

Once the defendant recovers somewhat from the shock of being sued, he or she will hire an attorney (assuming that the person would not choose to be a *pro se* litigant). The attorney will draft a *written answer* to the plaintiff's complaint and will file it with the clerk of the court in which the plaintiff initiated the suit. An answer to the complaint in Figure 2-9 is reproduced in Figure 2-10 for illustrative purposes. The defendant ordinarily is given a relatively short period of time to file an answer, usually thirty days. (The date-time-of-day stamp that was placed on the complaint by the clerk of the court lets the defendant know when the deadline for filing is.) The defendant's version of the incident giving rise to the suit is indicated in the answer. Also indicated is a summary of the *procedural reasons* why the defendant feels the plaintiff should not be awarded the remedy he or she is seeking (such as the plaintiff waited too long to initiate a suit because of the statute of limitations). If the defendant fails to file an answer by the deadline without having an extraordinarily good excuse, the plaintiff wins the suit.

In the period between when the defendant files his or her answer and the beginning of the trial, both the plaintiff and defendant gather evidence to support their contentions. Much of this evidence will be documented by the statements of persons who have knowledge that supports one or more of these contentions. The statements can be made under oath at the trial or under oath in writing prior to the

IN THE UNITED STATES DISTRICT COURT
FOR THE EASTERN DISTRICT OF TENNESSEE,
NORTHERN DIVISION

ELENA DeZAVALA a minor who)
sues by next friend and)
grandfather, LOUIS B. DeZAVALA,)
citizens and residents of)
Linn County, Iowa, and of no)
other place,)
)
            Plaintiffs)
)
)
    vs.)   No. 3-75-125
)
BETTY J. HOBBS and)
JAMES B. HOBBS,)
126 South Purdue Avenue,)
Oak Ridge, Anderson County,)
Tennessee,)
)
            Defendants)

C O M P L A I N T

    The plaintiff, Elena DeZavala, is a minor, nine years of age, who sues by next friend and grandfather, Louis B. DeZavala, both of whom are citizens and residents of Linn County, Iowa, and of no other place, and further aver that said plaintiff, Elena DeZavala, is the sole surviving child and lineal descendant and next of kin of Louis Victor DeZavala who died in Sullivan County, Tennessee on May 2, 1975. Said plaintiffs complain of the defendants, Betty J. Hobbs and James B. Hobbs, of 126 South Purdue Avenue, Oak Ridge, Tennessee, who are citizens and residents of Anderson County, Tennessee, and of no other place and State.

    Said plaintiff, Elena DeZavala, brings this suit by her grandfather and next friend, Louis B. DeZavala, by reason of the wrongful death of her father, Louis Victor DeZavala, who was divorced from the mother of the plaintiff, said mother having remarried.

FIGURE 2-9 A complaint. (Reprinted by permission from INTRODUCTION TO THE LEGAL SYSTEM, Second Edition by Bruce D. Fisher. Copyright © 1977 by West Publishing Company. All rights reserved.)

I

Plaintiff avers that the amount in controversy exceeds the sum of Ten Thousand Dollars ($10,000) exclusive of interest and costs, and that a complete diversity of citizenship exists between the plaintiff and the defendants, and jurisdiction of this Honorable Court is based on Title 28 U. S. Code Section 1332 (a).

II

Plaintiff avers that on May 2, 1975, at approximately 11:00 a.m., that the plaintiff's intestate-father was operating his vehicle in a southwardly direction along Interstate Highway 81, approximately one mile south of the intersection of said Interstate 81 with Tennessee Highway 137. Plaintiff avers that said vehicle of Louis Victor DeZavala was being operated in a southwardly direction in a proper and lawful manner upon its right hand side of said Interstate which at that point was a two lane two-way highway.

III

Plaintiff avers that said highway was plainly marked every thousand feet as a two-way highway for more than six miles in each direction from the location aforedescribed.

IV

Plaintiff avers that at said time and place as plaintiff's intestate and deceased father, Louis Victor DeZavala, was operating his said vehicle in a southwardly direction along said highway in a proper and lawful manner and upon its right hand side of the highway in broad daylight, that the defendant, Betty J. Hobbs, operating a vehicle within the purview of the Family Purpose Doctrine, which said vehicle was the property of her husband, James B. Hobbs, in a northwardly direction along said highway, meeting the automobile of the plaintiff's intestate. That the said **defendant, Betty J. Hobbs, while operating her automobile at**

-2-

FIGURE 2-9 (continued)

a high, reckless, wrongful and negligent rate of speed, and without keeping her said vehicle under control, and without keeping a lookout ahead, undertook to overtake and pass a truck traveling northwardly along said highway, and drove her said vehicle from its right hand or proper side of the highway to its left hand or improper side of the highway in an effort to overtake and pass said tractor-trailer traveling in the same direction in which she was traveling and drove her said vehicle in the manner and under the conditions aforedescribed into a violent head-on collision with the vehicle operated by the plaintiff's intestate and father.

V

Plaintiff avers that as the direct and proximate result of the negligence of the defendant as aforedescribed, operating her vehicle upon the highway upon the business of the defendant, James B. Hobbs, and within the purview of the Family Purpose Doctrine, that the plaintiff's intestate was crushed and mangled in a horrible manner sustaining such comprehensive, mangling and horrible injuries that as a direct and proximate result thereof after suffering a large amount of pain and mental anguish, that said plaintiff's intestate died, as a result of said injuries and as a proximate result of the negligence of the defendants as aforedescribed.

VI

Plaintiff avers that the defendants by the negligence as aforedescribed violated the following sections of the 1956 Tennessee Code Annotated, and that such violations on their part were the proximate contributing cause to the collision heretofore described and the death of plaintiff's intestate and the destruction of the automobile belonging to him at the time and place complained of:

FIGURE 2-9 (continued)

Section 59-815-Driving on right side of roadway.

Section 59-819-Limitations or overtaking on the left.

Section 59-820-(a) Further limitations on driving
to left of center of roadway.(1)

Section 59-821-No passing zones.

Section 59-823-Driving on roadways laned for traffic(a).

Section 59-852-Speed limit(a).

Section 59-858-Reckless driving(a).

VII

Plaintiff avers that the death of plaintiff's intestate resulted solely from the negligence of the defendants as aforedescribed and that the plaintiff's intestate was a young and healthy man, 30 years of age. Plaintiff was the intestate's only child. Plaintiff has further been put to the expense of the funeral bills and medical expenses, and the destruction of the automobile being occupied by the plaintiff's intestate at the time and place complained of.

WHEREFORE, plaintiff respectfully prays judgment against the defendants and each of them in the sum of Six Hundred Thousand Dollars ($600,000) and respectfully demand a jury to try the issues joined.

KENNERLY, MONTGOMERY, HOWARD & FINLEY

By _____
George D. Montgomery,
Attorneys for Plaintiff
12th Floor
Bank of Knoxville Building
Post Office Box 442
Knoxville, Tennessee 37901

1/5

COST BOND

We do hereby acknowledge ourselves as surety for the costs in this cause in an amount not to exceed Two Hundred Fifty Dollars ($250).

KENNERLY, MONTGOMERY, HOWARD & FINLEY

By _____

FIGURE 2-9 (continued)

IN THE UNITED STATES DISTRICT COURT
FOR THE EASTERN DISTRICT OF TENNESSEE,
NORTHERN DIVISION

ELENA DeZAVALA b/n/f
LOUIS B. DeZAVALA,

        Plaintiffs

VS

BETTY J. HOBBS and
JAMES B. HOBBS,

        Defendants

NO. 3-75-125

FILED JUN 18 1975

ANSWER

    The defendants, Betty J. Hobbs and James B. Hobbs, for answer to the complaint filed against them in this cause, say as follows:

    1. They admit that they are citizens of Tennessee and that Louis Victor DeZavala died in Sullivan County, Tennessee, on May 2, 1975, but they have no knowledge as to the other allegations in the first and second paragraphs of the complaint so they neither admit nor deny such allegations and demand strict proof thereof.

    2. They admit that this Court has jurisdiction of this action, provided there is diversity of citizenship, as alleged.

    3. They admit that the defendant, Betty J. Hobbs, was driving the automobile which collided with the automobile driven by the deceased, Louis Victor DeZavala at or about the time and place alleged.

    4. They admit that the defendant, James B. Hobbs, was the owner of the automobile being driven by his wife, Betty J. Hobbs, at the time of this accident, and that the family purpose doctrine is applicable.

FIGURE 2-10 The answer to the complaint in Figure 2-9. (Reprinted by permission from IN-TRODUCTION TO THE LEGAL SYSTEM, Second Edition by Bruce D. Fisher. Copyright © 1977 by West Publishing Company. All rights reserved.)

5. They deny all allegations of negligence and statutory violations on the part of the defendant, Betty J. Hobbs.

6. They admit that the deceased, Louis Victor DeZavala, died as a result of injuries in this accident, but they aver that his death was instantaneous.

7. For lack of knowledge, they neither admit nor deny the allegations in paragraph VII of the complaint, and demand strict proof thereof.

8. They plead proximate or remote contributory negligence on the part of the deceased.

AND NOW HAVING ANSWERED, the defendants pray to be hence dismissed with their costs and demand a jury to try this cause.

Fred H. Cagle, Jr.
P. O. Box 39
Knoxville, Tennessee 37901

Attorney for Defendants

FRANTZ, McCONNELL & SEYMOUR

Of Counsel

CERTIFICATE OF SERVICE

I certify that an exact copy of the foregoing document has been served upon counsel for all parties to the litigation to which it pertains, either by hand delivery of a copy thereof to the offices of said counsel, or by mailing a copy to said counsel in a properly addressed and stamped envelope regularly deposited in the United States Mail.

This 17 day of Jan, 1975.

For FRANTZ, McCONNELL & SEYMOUR

FIGURE 2-10 (continued)

trial. Statements of the latter type are referred to as *depositions.* They can be solicited by either the attorney for the plaintiff or the attorney for the defendant. An attorney may choose to document the evidence in a witness's statement by a pretrial deposition for any of several reasons—for example, the witness will be unavailable for the trial or the attorney wants to obtain a statement of the relevant information while it is still fresh in the witness's mind.

Prior to the trial each party to the lawsuit usually has an opportunity to find out, or *discover,* the sorts of evidence the other party has and is likely to use. Also prior to the trial the attorneys for the plaintiff and defendant may have a conference with the judge who will be presiding at the trial. In it each side will indicate what it will attempt to prove and how it will attempt to prove it. Such conferences can reduce trial time because they can pinpoint what each side would have to prove in order to win the suit. Such conferences also could demonstrate to the defendant that he or she would have little or no chance of winning the suit and could thereby motivate the defendant to try to reach an out-of-court settlement with the plaintiff. Or they could demonstrate to the plaintiff that he or she would have little or no chance of being awarded the remedy being sought from the court and could thereby motivate the plaintiff to drop the suit. Out-of-court settlements are desirable because they save both parties to a suit the expense and emotional strain of a trial. Such settlements also are desirable from the court's point of view. Most courts are overloaded with cases, and as a result a relatively long period of time often elapses between the initiation of a suit and the trial.

If the plaintiff and defendant are unable to settle their dispute before their suit is scheduled to be tried, they will become participants in a complex competitive team game known as a *trial.* The arena for the game is a *courtroom.* The main participants, beside the plaintiff and defendant, will be their attorneys, their witnesses, the judge, and the jury. The plaintiff and defendant *may* agree to play the game without a jury, in which case the judge will assume the jury's functions.

There are two teams. One consists of the plaintiff, his or her attorney (or attorneys), and witnesses. The other consists of the defendant, his or her attorney (or attorneys), and witnesses whose testimony can be helpful to the defendant.

The *judge* decides which team wins the game; and, if it is the plaintiff's team, what the prize—the judicial remedy—should be. The judge also functions as a *referee* and sees to it that both teams obey the rules of the game. The judge settles disputes when one team charges the other with violating a rule (or rules) and as referee enforces the rules of the game in an *appropriate* and *evenhanded* manner. If the judge fails to enforce the rules in such a manner and the decision is appealed to a higher, or *appellate,* court, it can be reversed on this basis. Obviously, the team that lost the game would be the one to attempt to demonstrate that the rules were not enforced in an appropriate and evenhanded manner. The team that won would be unlikely to question the enforcement of the rules, even if they felt the judge did it in a blatantly inappropriate or unevenhanded manner.

A judge is a human being and like other human beings can make mistakes and be biased. A person becomes a judge either by being appointed or being elected. If

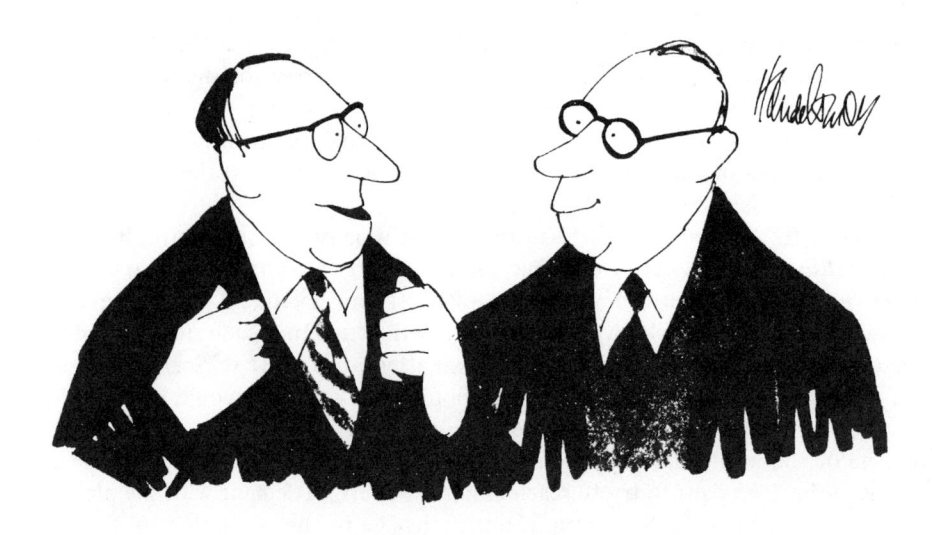

"This daily metamorphosis never fails to amaze me. Around the house, I'm a perfect idiot. I come to court, put on a black robe, and, by God, I'm it!" *

Drawing by Handelsman; Copyright 1971, THE NEW YORKER MAGAZINE, INC.

the means was appointment it could have been primarily for political reasons. If he or she was elected, it could have been primarily on the basis of the "image" he or she communicated to the voters. While the *office of judge* certainly should be respected, a person holding that office should not be regarded as superhuman.

The *jury* in a civil case assists the judge in deciding questions of fact. The plaintiff and defendant are apt to present different versions of what happened. The function of the jury is to decide who is most likely to be telling the truth. They are supposed to weigh the evidence presented by each party to support its position on each question of fact and then to decide which position is best supported by the evidence. The jury bases its decision on what is presented. If the attorney for one party does not adequately present the evidence that supports his or her client's position, the client could lose the suit on this basis. Hence, the relative competency of the attorneys representing the parties can have a significant impact on who wins.

The verdict rendered by a jury in a civil suit does not have to be accepted by the judge, at least theoretically (Fisher, 1977). If a jury renders a verdict that is completely at odds with the evidence, a party who would be hurt by such a decision can ask the court for *judgment notwithstanding the verdict*. If the judge agrees that the verdict was not consistent with the evidence, he or she can disregard it and decide in favor of the moving party. Of course, the judge's decision would be likely to be appealed by the party in whose favor the jury rendered their verdict.

The attorneys representing the parties to a lawsuit can be viewed as team captains and coaches. If the parties do not choose to be *pro se* litigants, they will empower an attorney to present their case to the judge and jury—that is, to speak for them. A litigant retains the right, however, to discharge his or her attorney at any point in the proceedings if dissatisfied with how the case is being presented. The attorney representing each party assumes the major responsibility for the planning and presentation of the client's case (and thus functions as the captain of the client's team). The attorney coaches the witnesses who will provide evidence to support his or her client's case. Attorneys are ethically bound when functioning in this latter role not to encourage witnesses to lie, or *perjure* themselves. Their primary responsibility is to present the strongest case they can to support their client's position in the suit and to make certain that the manner in which the court proceedings are conducted by the judge does not violate their client's constitutional guarantees of *procedural due process.*

The witnesses an attorney uses to support a client's case are of two types. The first consists of persons having *direct knowledge* of some aspect of the action giving rise to the suit whose *testimony* would be expected to provide evidence that supports one or more aspects of a client's case. Such testimony usually consists of a description of what the witness heard and/or saw. (It also may include a description of what he smelled, touched, or tasted.)

The second type is referred to as an *expert witness.* Those functioning in this role are usually licensed or certified as competent to engage in a profession such as medicine, clinical psychology, speech-language pathology, or audiology. Because of their training and experience in a particular discipline, they can be viewed as experts whose judgments on matters relevant to that discipline are likely to be accurate enough that they are admissible as evidence. A speech-language pathologist, for example, might be asked to evaluate an aphasic and to testify (give an expert opinion) whether the person was able to communicate well enough to continue to manage his or her financial affairs. An audiologist might be asked to evaluate a factory worker who developed a presumably job-related, noise-induced hearing loss and to give an expert opinion as to how much the worker was handicapped by it. Such testimony could assist a worker's compensation court in deciding how much to award. The expert witness is dealt with further in Chapter 11.

Now that the roles of the participants in the game (trial) have been described, we will consider the rules. The civil trial game consists of a series of events, or activities, that are ordered in a particular manner. These will be summarized here. (The primary source for the information presented in this discussion was Grilliot, 1979, pp. 245-271.)

The first event or activity in a civil trial is the selection of the *jury.* The members of a jury are selected from a pool of people who usually are registered voters from the community in which the court is located. They were told to be at the courthouse and available for jury duty.

At the beginning of the selection process, a group of prospective jurors are questioned by the attorneys for both parties and by the judge. The purpose of the questioning is to determine whether there are grounds for believing that any of them are unlikely to be *impartial* (without prejudice or bias) when rendering a verdict. The attorneys for both parties can challenge the potential impartiality of as many as they wish, and those that the judge agrees are apt to be biased or prejudiced will be replaced. In addition, each party is given a limited number of *peremptory challenges*. These can be used to remove prospective jurors without having to show cause. As prospective jurors are removed through successful challenges, they are replaced with others from the pool. The examination-replacement process continues until an adequate number have been selected to form a jury. The jury members are then sworn in.

Both parties to a lawsuit are seeking to form a jury that *at the very least* could be expected to be impartial and *ideally* would tend to be biased in favor of their case. The attorneys for both sides should have in mind the profile for such a jury when engaging in the selection process. By using challenges (particularly peremptory challenges) wisely, each will attempt to form a jury the profile of which will approximate his or her ideal one as closely as possible. Obviously, if one party's attorney were more knowledgeable than the other's about the attributes of jurors who would be most likely to believe his or her client, the resulting jury would be more likely to be sympathetic to one side than to the other. Thus, it is possible (but not probable) for the winner to be determined on the first move of the game (trial).

The next event that occurs in a civil trial is the *opening statements* of the plaintiff's and defendant's attorneys. The plaintiff's attorney, in an opening statement, explains the facts of the case to the judge and jury from his or her client's perspective, including an explanation of the *legal theory* that would warrant the court's awarding the remedy that is sought. The attorney also indicates what he or she intends to prove during the trial. If the defendant's attorney chooses to make an opening statement, it will deal with these topics from his or her client's perspective. The attorneys for both parties, through their opening statements, are attempting to develop attitudes in the judge and jury that would cause them to believe their client's case. This task would be easier for one side than the other if the jury were not truly impartial.

Following completion of the opening statements, the attorney for the plaintiff presents his or her client's case. To win the suit and be awarded the remedy, the plaintiff must present *evidence* to prove those *allegations* made in the complaint that are disputed by the defendant. Admissible evidence would include relevant documents, fact testimony from witnesses, and opinion testimony from expert witnesses. If an ordinary witness (i.e., not an expert who has documents or knowledge of facts that would support the plaintiff's case) refuses to voluntarily surrender the documents or testify, he or she can be ordered to do so by the court (judge). The court wold issue an order referred to as a *subpoena*. If a witness disregards the subpoena, he or she can be punished for *contempt of court*.

The defendant's attorney will attempt to *discredit* (or refute) the evidence presented by the plaintiff's attorney. If the defendant's attorney is successful, the plaintiff *should* lose the suit. (Unfortunately, good guys sometimes lose in courts of law.) The defendant's attorney will question the relevance and credibility of the documents the plaintiff's attorney introduces, the interpretation that is being given to them, or both. The defendant's attorney will *cross-examine* the plaintiff's "fact" witnesses in an attempt to raise questions about the credibility of their testimony in the minds of the judge and members of the jury and will also cross-examine the plaintiff's witnesses (if any) in an attempt to cast doubt on the credibility of their opinions. The defense attorney may even produce expert witnesses who will question the validity of the opinions of the plaintiff's expert witnesses. While perhaps unable to prove that the opinions of the defendant's experts are more credible than those of the plaintiff's, the defendant's attorney can at least suggest to the judge and jury that experts disagree and, hence, little weight should be given to the testimony of the plaintiff's expert witnesses.

After the plaintiff's presentation has been made, the defendant's attorney may ask the judge for an *involuntary dismissal* of the suit on the grounds that the plaintiff failed to prove the allegations in the complaint. If the judge agrees to grant this motion, the trial ends and the plaintiff loses. If the judge refuses to grant it, the trial continues.

The attorney for the defendant will attempt to prove the allegations he or she made in *answer* to the plaintiff's complaint by presenting evidence. He or she will use the same types of evidence as did the plaintiff's attorney, including documents, fact witnesses, and expert witnesses. The attorney for the plaintiff will have an opportunity to cross-examine defense witnesses and challenge the credibility of the documents introduced as evidence.

After the defendant's presentation has been completed, the plaintiff's attorney has an opportunity to *rebut* the defendant's case. This ordinarily is the plaintiff's last opportunity to introduce new evidence.

After the plaintiff completes the rebuttal, the defendant is given an opportunity for a *rejoinder* to attempt to refute any new evidence introduced by the plaintiff's attorney during the rebuttal. This ordinarily is the defendant's last opportunity to introduce new evidence.

At this point in the trial (or at any future point prior to the case's being submitted to the jury) either party may make a motion for a *directed verdict.* When *plaintiffs* make this motion, they are indicating that they feel their case is so strong that no reasonable jury could decide against them. When defendants make this motion, they are indicating that they feel the plaintiff's case has no merit. If the judge grants the motion, the moving party will win the suit without its being submitted to the jury. Obviously, a judge would be unlikely to grant a motion for a directed verdict unless the case for granting the motion was extremely strong. The party that lost the suit probably could appeal the decision on this basis, and if the judge could not justify granting the motion, the decision would be likely to be reversed by the *appellate* court reviewing it. If the judge refuses to grant the motion for a directed verdict, the trial continues.

Both parties now have what will ordinarily be their last opportunity to convince the judge and jury (particularly the latter) of the merits of their cases by presenting their *closing arguments*. The plaintiff's attorney presents closing arguments first, but he or she may reserve some time for a rebuttal following the defendant's closing arguments. Both attorneys will summarize their cases and will indicate to the jury why they should reach the verdict desired by their clients.

Following the completion of closing arguments, the suit is ready to be presented to the jury. Before the jury begins its deliberations, the judge gives the jurors instructions. He or she summarizes the case, explains the substantive law that applies to it, and indicates what type of verdict is desired—general or special. If a *general verdict* is requested, the jury will decide who won the suit. If they decide for a plaintiff who is seeking damages, they also may make a recommendation concerning the amount of damages to be awarded. If the judge requests a *special verdict,* the jury will answer certain questions pertaining to facts on which the parties to the suit do not agree. The *facts* generated by the jury in its answers to these questions will be incorporated by the judge into the decision. How the judge words the questions, obviously, can influence the jury's answers and thereby the ultimate outcome of the case. The general verdict is preferred by many legal scholars for this reason.

After being instructed by the judge, the jury will leave the courtroom and *begin its deliberation.* It will continue its deliberation until its members are able to reach agreement on a verdict or until it becomes obvious that they will be unable to do so. Once the jury has reached a verdict, the leader presents it in writing to the judge who, in turn, informs both parties to the suit.

At this point—that is, before the judge renders judgment—the attorney for the party who would lose the suit if the jury's verdict were adhered to may file a motion to have the verdict set aside (i.e., a motion for a *judgment notwithstanding the verdict of the jury*) or for a new trial. A judge would be unlikely to grant either motion unless there was clearly something wrong with the manner in which the jury reached its verdict. If, for example, one or more members of the jury were coerced into voting in a particular way, this could be grounds for a judge to grant a request for a new trial.

If the judge refused to grant a motion for a new trial or for a judgment notwithstanding the verdict of the jury or if no such motions were made, he or she would at this point in the proceedings *render judgment* by declaring in writing who won the suit and, if the winner was the plaintiff, by indicating the remedy being awarded—that is, indicating what the defendant is ordered to do or to refrain from doing. If the defendant does not voluntarily do what is ordered by the judge (e.g., pay damages), the plaintiff can seek an *order of execution* to force the defendant to do it. The *judgment,* or court decision, for the suit initiated by the complaint in Figure 2-9 is reproduced for illustrative purposes in Figure 2-11.

The party losing the suit can appeal the judgment to an appellate court if dissatisfied with it. If the case were tried in a federal court, the appeal would be made to the U.S. Court of Appeals. If it were tried in a state court, the appeal would be made to the intermediate appellate court in that state court system. The party initiating the appeal would claim that *procedural errors* were made by the

JUDGMENT ON JURY VERDICT   CIV 31 (7-63)

United States District Court

FOR THE
EASTERN DISTRICT OF TENNESSEE, NORTHERN DIVISION

ELENA DEZAVALA, b/n/f
and grandfather
LOUIS B. DEZAVALA

      vs.

BETTY J. HOBBS &
JAMES HOBBS

CIVIL ACTION FILE NO. 3-75-125

JUDGMENT

This action came on for trial before the Court and a jury, Honorable Robert L. Taylor, United States District Judge, presiding, and the issues having been duly tried and the jury having duly rendered its verdict,

It is Ordered and Adjudged that the Plaintiffs, Elena Dezavala, b/n/f and grandfather, Louis B. Dezavala, recover of the defendants Betty J. Hobbs and James Hobbs, the sum of Twenty-five Thousand ($25,000) Dollars, plus property damage in the amount of Three Hundred ($300) Dollars, with interest thereon at the rate of six percent as provided by law, and their costs of action.

Dated at Knoxville, Tennessee , this 25th day of August , 19 75.

KARL D. SAULPAW, JR.
Clerk of Court

By *Jean Medlock*

Filed 25 day of Aug 1975
Ent'd Order Book 71, p. 326
KARL D. SAULPAW, JR., CLERK
by *Jean Medlock* Dep. Clerk

FIGURE 2-11 The court decision. (Reprinted by permission from INTRODUCTION TO THE LEGAL SYSTEM, Second Edition by Bruce D. Fisher. Copyright © 1977 by West Publishing Company. All rights reserved.)

court (particularly the judge) during the trial. If the justices of the appellate court agreed to review the case, they would examine a transcript of the courtroom proceedings to determine whether the proper legal rules had been applied. If they detect an error (or errors) that could have affected the outcome, they are likely to reverse the decision of the trial court and order it to retry the case, applying the correct procedures. If the appellate court affirms the trial court decision, the party *may* be able to appeal the trial court judgment to higher appellate courts, including the U.S. Supreme Court.

The legal fees for any appellate court appeal can be high. Those losing a suit may decide against appealing the court decision even if they feel there are excellent grounds for doing so because of the expense involved.

A court judgment ordinarily is not carried out until the appeal process has been completed. A defendant losing a suit who wishes to delay having to comply with the court judgment can do so by making all possible appeals. A corporation or governmental unit that loses a suit in which it was the defendant may use such a strategy. Since such an organization is likely to employ its own attorneys, the costs involved in doing so may not be high enough to outweigh the advantages of delaying implementation of the court decision.

The Administrative Hearing

Speech-language pathologists and audiologists (particularly the former) are more likely to become involved in administrative hearings than in civil suits. They may be asked to testify as ordinary or expert witnesses at a hearing instigated by the parents of a child who has a communicative disorder in which they are seeking to force the school system to modify the child's program in a way that they feel would more adequately meet the child's special educational needs. Such hearings (referred to as *due process hearings*) may be held to enforce provisions of P.L. 94-142 (Downey, 1980a, 1980b), which includes forcing school systems to provide "a free, appropriate public education in the least restrictive environment" for all children for whom they are responsible. (For further information about this law, see Appendix C.)

Administrative hearings are conducted under the auspices of an administrative agency. With respect to the due process hearings that are a component of the enforcement mechanism for P.L. 94-142, the administrative agency under whose auspices such hearings are conducted is the public school district.

An administrative hearing can be a means to an end or an end in itself. It can be a means for resolving issues in dispute or it can be a step in a process that terminates with the initiation of a civil suit. Ideally, most of the disputes dealt with in such hearings will be resolved at this level rather than having to be decided in the court system.

An administrative hearing tends to be a more economical means of settling a dispute than a court trial for several reasons. First, a *hearing officer* rather than a judge presides. A hearing officer typically is neither a judge nor an attorney. He or she is supposed to be a *neutral person* (i.e., not an employee of the agency under whose auspices the hearing is being held and with no personal or professional interests that could conflict with his or her objectivity) who has expertise on the issues under dispute and knows how to conduct a hearing. (He or she would probably have learned how to conduct a hearing by attending a workshop for prospective hearing officers sponsored by the agency under whose auspices he or she would conduct hearings if requested.) Responsibilities of a hearing officer can be summarized as follows:

> A hearing officer at an administrative hearing is charged with the duty of insuring that: the hearing is conducted in an orderly and concise fashion, parties are able to present witnesses who have relevant testimony, relevant evidence is introduced into the record, and rulings are made on objections posed by parties during the course of the hearing. The hearing officer assumes these duties in order to assure that parties are afforded procedural due process and to assure that a clear and concise record (transcripts plus exhibits) of the hearing is created. A transcript which is clear and intelligible is essential because such a transcript serves as an aid to the hearing officer in the writing of his report and, should appeal be taken . . . serves as the basis for the . . . ruling on the merits of the appeal. (Reprinted from unpublished material used by the Wisconsin Department of Public Instruction for training hearing officers)

A second reason why an administrative hearing tends to be more economical than a trial is that a jury is not used. A hearing officer assumes the responsibilities of both judge and jury in a civil suit.

A third reason why an administrative hearing tends to be more economical than a trial is that the arena in which it is conducted is an ordinary conference room. Also the hearing officer (partially because of where hearings are conducted) swears in witnesses and performs other functions that ordinarily are performed by court personnel during a trial.

An adminstrative hearing is a legal forum conducted by rules quite similar to those used for conducting a civil trial. All testimony is given under oath. Both parties have the right to cross-examine each other's witnesses and to attempt to refute each other's documentary evidence. Both parties have the right to be represented by an attorney. Both parties have the right to *subpoena* documentary evidence and the testimony of reluctant witnesses. And the entire proceedings ordinarily are recorded, either by an audiotape recorder or a court stenographer.

The structure of an administrative hearing tends to be quite similar to that of a civil trial. Both parties begin by presenting opening statements in which they summarize the allegations they will attempt to prove. Following this, each party presents its case—that is, the evidence supporting its allegations, which could include documents and the testimony of ordinary and expert witnesses. The parties are then given an opportunity to present rebuttal evidence following which they make their closing statements.

When closing the hearing the hearing officer usually specifies the date by which he or she will present a copy of the *written decision* to the parties. The party against whom he decides can appeal the decision. In some instances the first level of appeal will be within the agency under whose auspices the hearing was conducted; in others it will be in the courts. (For further information about the structure of administrative hearings, see Downey, 1980a, 1980b.)

REFERENCES

BLACK, H. C., *Black's Law Dictionary* (Rev. 4th Ed.). St. Paul, Minn.: West Publishing Company (1968).

DAVID, K. C., *Administrative Law: Cases-Text-Problems*. St. Paul, Minn.: West Publishing Company (1977).

Digest of State Laws and Regulations for School Language, Speech, and Hearing Programs. Washington, D.C.: American Speech and Hearing Association (1973).

DOWNEY, M., Conduct of the due process hearing. *Asha*, 22, 332-333 (1980a).

DOWNEY, M., Due process hearings and PL 94-142. *Asha*, 22, 255-257 (1980b).

DOWNEY, M., Legal developments—Antitrust and sunset laws. *Asha*, 21, 7-11 (1979).

FISHER, B. D., *Introduction to the Legal System* (2nd Ed.). St. Paul, Minn.: West Publishing Company (1977).

GIFIS, S. H., *Law Dictionary*. Woodbury, N.Y.: Barron's Educational Service (1975).

GRILLIOT, H. J., *Introduction to Law and the Legal System* (2nd Ed.). Boston: Houghton Mifflin (1979).

JOHNSON, W., *People in Quandaries*. New York: Harper & Row (1946).

KORZYBSKI, A., *Science and Sanity*. Lakeville, Conn.: Institute of General Semantics (1933).

ROMBAUER, M. D., *Legal Problem Solving*. St. Paul, Minn.: West Publishing Company (1978).

3

Licensure, Certification, Registration, and Accreditation

One of the ways by which our legal system directly and indirectly influences the clinical functioning of speech-language pathologists and audiologists is through the mechanisms of licensure, certification, registration, and accreditation. These set limits on the *client populations* to whom a person certified or licensed as a speech-language pathologist or audiologist may provide services and on the *services* that he or she may provide to persons in these populations. A person certified or licensed as an audiologist probably would be permitted to provide certain services to certain populations (e.g., fitting hearing aids to persons who have severe hearing losses) that a person certified or licensed as a speech-language pathologist would not ordinarily be permitted to provide and vice versa. Licensure and certification also set limits on *how services can be provided* by requiring adherence to a code of ethics. Failure to function in a manner consistent with the code of ethics can result in one's license being revoked or one's certification being taken away. In addition, licensure and certification impose restrictions on how practitioners are *trained*. The requirements for the Certificate of Clinical Competence in Speech-Language Pathology and the Certificate of Clinical Competence in Audiology awarded by the American Speech-Language-Hearing Association and those for state licensure (both public school and general) influence the curriculums of speech-language pathology and audiology training programs. Finally, licensure and certification requirements can influence how speech-language pathologists and audiologists are *paid for their services*. Many federal health insurance programs such as Medicare stipulate that to be covered speech-language pathology services must be provided by a practitioner who has met the academic and practicum requirements for the Certificate of Clinical Competence in Speech-Language Pathology. Also, if a school district wishes to be partially reimbursed by the state for services provided communicatively handicapped children, the services must be provided by speech-language pathologists who are credentialed by the state department of education.

WHAT IS THE MOTIVATION FOR INITIATING LICENSURE, CERTIFICATION, REGISTRATION, AND ACCREDITATION?

Whenever individuals or groups decide to attempt to change the status quo, it is almost always because they expect to derive some benefit from doing so. Their expectations may or may not be realistic. But so long as they believe they will benefit from a change, they are likely to attempt to bring it about. The reason or reasons that they give for wanting to change the status quo may not be the real reasons or may not be all of the reasons. Rather, they are apt to be reasons they feel would be *acceptable* to persons who must approve the change.

The regulation of professionals through licensure, certification, accreditation, and registration is a relatively recent phenomenon. In the health field it appears to have begun with medicine; many states attempted to regulate medical practice prior to 1800. It was not until just before the Civil War, however, that interest in regulating health professionals reached a national level with the establishment of the American Medical Association in 1847 and the American Dental Association in 1859 (Levine, 1978). Most other health-related fields were not regulated prior to the twentieth century.

The individuals and groups who seek regulation of an occupation (particularly a profession) tend to be those who are members of it rather than consumers of its services. The process that must be undertaken to achieve some form of regulation is ordinarily quite expensive—both in financial cost and time invested. Since regulation would be likely to place restrictions on the activities of the persons seeking it, why would they be motivated to invest their time and money to pursue it? What *benefits* would they expect to receive from regulation of their occupation? I will attempt in this section to provide a partial answer to these questions.

The primary justification that usually is given for regulating an occupation is the *protection of public health, safety, or morals.* Those seeking regulation argue that without it,

> incompetent practitioners will offer their services. Prospective buyers of these services are said not to be able to distinguish between qualified and unqualified persons, and this is considered to be especially true if consumers buy services of the particular kind only at infrequent intervals. Where the consequences of the employment of unqualified persons can be expected to be seriously adversive to the purchaser, and especially where the conse-

> quences of incompetently rendered service are irreversible, it is thought to be desirable that . . . some examining or other procedure [be administered] to determine who are qualified to practice, and prevent those who are unqualified from offering their services. The average quality of those permitted to practice is raised, and by the exclusion of "quacks" and incompetents the public is protected from the error of employing them. (Rottenberg, 1968, p. 283)

Though these arguments were formulated to justify licensing, they have been used to justify other forms of regulation as well.

Although regulation can be justified on the basis that it tends to *raise the average quality* of the services offered by the members of a profession, this may not be the primary reason why members are motivated to pursue it. Their primary reason may be to gain *legal status,* or recognition, for the profession:

> Once a profession is awarded legal status and is given the exclusive right to practice in the field of its competence, it can inhibit the practice of imposters by taking action in the courts. . . . Each profession defines an area of practice in which it has a monopoly and fights hard to preserve that unique area. (Lum, 1978, p. 156)

Thus, by gaining legal status through regulation a health profession can establish what its members hope will be an *exclusive claim to a segment of the health service territory.* The total territory consists of all services for preventing and ameliorating the mental-physical disorders that a human being can develop; each profession is seeking to be granted the exclusive right to provide *certain* of these services to persons having *certain* mental-physical disorders. If they are successful, they will have a *monopoly* (or close to a monopoly) on the delivery of services included in the segment of the territory to which they have staked a claim. Medicine is an example of a profession that has been successful in establishing a near monopoly on the delivery of services in a segment of this territory.

When a profession is awarded a monopoly, or near monopoly, with respect to the delivery of certain services, it is expected to see to it that these services are provided in a responsible manner. According to Lum,

> Society accords a monopoly to a profession with respect to its practice and standard setting on the premise that no lay person understands esoteric knowledge on which the profession rests, and therefore no lay person can judge what should be done. Society allows a profession to hold a monopoly because it is convinced that the profession is dedicated to an ethical or altruistic ideal in serving society. Society continues to allow this monopoly as long as it is convinced that a profession is exercising its privileges responsibly and aids and/or serves its clientele without exploitation.
>
> Under its monopoly, a profession has the purpose of protecting not only the society it serves, but also its members, making it possible for them to practice effectively. Its protection, which occurs through methods passed on by socialization, takes different form as the profession confronts internal as well as external dangers.

Internally, a profession must protect society and its members against the incompetent or dishonest member whose actions may damage trust in the profession. A profession controls the number and kinds of persons who are allowed to enter and to study through the establishment of admission criteria and determining the length and types of programs allowed. These controls are imposed in order to prevent incompetent persons from entering the profession and to avoid an oversupply of practitioners as well. In addition, it controls the body of knowledge on which the practice rests and maintains the quality and standards of its education through a process of external accreditation. It further controls admission to the profession through licensing procedures as well as through various certification and credential procedures. It opposes efforts to establish conditions that would make its practice difficult or impossible. Each profession has an obligation to police its own ranks and make certain that those who wear the name and display the license are in fact ethical and competent practitioners. From this obligation stem efforts to enforce the code of ethics of the profession even to the extent of expelling members who flagrantly violate provisions of its code. Thus, a physician can have his license revoked or a lawyer can be "disbarred." Professional associations aid practitioners in obtaining legal sanction for their monopoly. (Lum, 1978, pp. 155-156)

In a sense, when a profession is granted a monopoly, it enters into a *contract* with the community that granted it. As compensation for the legal status accorded it, the members of the profession agree to provide certain services that are of an *acceptable quality*. If they fail to do what they promised, the community has the right (perhaps even the obligation) to terminate their monopoly as providers of these services.

One possible result of regulating the practice of a profession is reducing the number of persons entering it. The higher the cost for a new person to qualify as a practitioner, the less likely such persons are to attempt to qualify (particularly if they do not expect the financial rewards of qualifying to be worth the effort). Several factors are likely to contribute to the cost of entering a profession. Perhaps the most obvious one is the cost of the training or education required for entering it. In addition to the direct cost associated with this education or training, there is also an indirect cost—the money the person would have earned if he or she had worked instead of pursuing the necessary schooling.

Another cost associated with entering a profession is the investment of time and energy required to gain the knowledge and experience necessary to be licensed or certified. When the members of a professional group are proposing licensing or certification requirements it is not uncommon for them to make these requirements *more demanding* than those they were required to satisfy, and if their recommendations are accepted, to award themselves the new (or revised) license or certificate through a *grandfather clause*. Such clauses stipulate "that those who have already entered and are practicing the occupation be qualified *pro forma* and exempted from examination" (Rottenberg, 1968, p. 283). The term *pro forma* in this context is used to suggest that the license or certificate is awarded not on the basis of a conviction that those awarded it under the grandfather clause are qualified but merely to facilitate acceptance of the license or certificate by existing practitioners. A person would be unlikely to support a change in requirements for certification or licensure if its adoption means that he or she would no longer qualify for certification or licensure.

HOW ARE OCCUPATIONS REGULATED?

A number of approaches are used to regulate the entrance of new practitioners into an occupation (see Figure 3-1). Some are initiated and administered by a professional organization, and others are administered by a governmental agency. Each of these is described in this section and the advantages and disadvantages are indicated.

Types of Regulation Administered by a Professional Organization

A professional organization can regulate the practice of an occupation in two main ways: through *certification* and *accreditation*. Both are used by the American Speech-Language-Hearing Association to regulate the practice of speech-language pathology and audiology by persons or agencies who wish to be regulated.

Certification Certification is "a voluntary mechanism by which a nongovernmental agency or association grants recognition to an individual who has met certain predetermined qualifications specified by that agency or association"

FIGURE 3-1 Approaches used for occupational regulation in health-related fields.

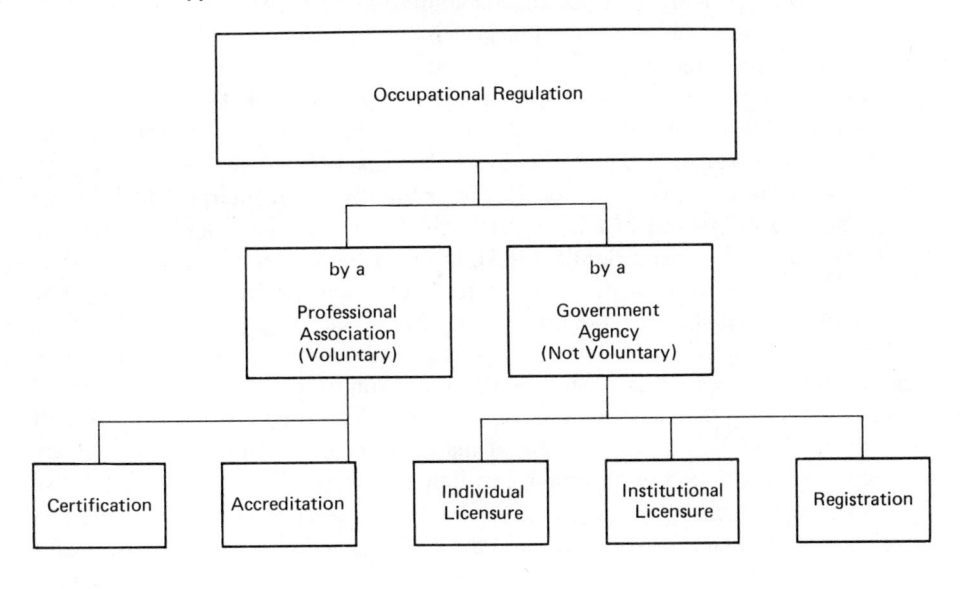

(Roemer, 1974, p. 26). Because certification is a *voluntary* mechanism, persons who are not certified in an occupation can *legally* enter it (assuming that no license is required). They may, however, have difficulty finding employment because employers may discriminate against those who do not possess the certification. There are several reasons why employers are likely to do this. First, it simplifies the hiring process. The person doing the hiring can avoid having to evaluate the competency of each applicant by insisting on possession of the appropriate certification. Its possession by an applicant signifies to the employer that the applicant's education and experience have been adequate to meet at least minimum performance standards. Second, it may simplify the process for obtaining payment from *third parties* (such as private and government-sponsored insurance programs) for clinical services. Third parties usually stipulate that they will only pay for services that are provided by persons whom they regard as qualified practitioners. Almost all such providers would consider a person who was certified as competent by the national association to which members of the profession belong to be a qualified practitioner. (An example of such an association would be the American Speech-Language-Hearing Association.)

Certification may be offered to acknowledge either *basic* or *specialty* qualifications. When all states regulate the practice of a profession on a basic level through licensure (as is the case in medicine), then professional organizations tend to concentrate their efforts on *specialty certification*. (A specialty for which certification is offered in medicine is otolaryngology.) If all states were to regulate the practice of speech-language pathology and audiology through licensure, the American Speech-Language-Hearing Association would be likely to emphasize specialty certification rather than its present certification program (Governmental regulation, 1969). A specialty for which certification could be offered in speech-language pathology is habilitation and rehabilitation with augmentative communication systems (Position paper on nonspeech communication, 1981) and in audiology is aural rehabilitation.

Certification can be offered for a relatively *narrow* subject matter specialty, such as administering and interpreting a test or using a specific intervention approach, or for a relatively broad one. Tests that practitioners in the field of communicative disorders have been certified to administer and interpret include the *Porch Index of Communicative Ability* (Porch, 1967) and the *Staggered Spondaic Word Test* (Katz, Basil, and Smith, 1963). Intervention strategies that practitioners in the field of communicative disorders have been certified to use include Blissymbolics augmentative communication (Kates, McNaughton, and Silverman, no date) and the *Hollins Precision Fluency Shaping Program* (Webster, 1974). While organizations that award this type of certification cannot legally prevent uncertified persons from using their tests or intervention strategies, they can make it difficult for them to do so by making full sets of materials available only to those who are certified or in the process of becoming certified.

Most professional certification programs have several components in addition to requiring acceptance of a code of ethics. First, they require the successful completion of one or more courses that may or may not be offered for academic credit by a college or university. Second, they require a specified minimum amount of supervised practical (practicum) experience. Third, they may require an internship following completion of the academic and practicum requirements. Fourth, they may require the passing of an examination. And fifth, they may require persons who have the certification to expose themselves periodically to continuing education. (The words *expose themselves* were used because most continuing education courses do not have examinations or other mechanisms for determining how much a participant has learned.) The American Speech-Language-Hearing Association's certificates of clinical competence in speech-language pathology and in audiology require the first four of these components. The fifth is encouraged and is likely to become mandatory.

While certification encourages practitioners to obtain the training necessary to perform their services competently and to behave ethically in their interactions with others, it has several limitations as a mechanism for insuring competence. According to Roemer,

> The basic requirement for certification is completion of an approved educational program, but the multiplicity of educational programs in different settings for the same occupation makes surveillance difficult. For many health occupations, no substitution of work experience or recognition of equivalent qualifications is allowed in place of academic qualifications for certification. Very few certifying bodies use examinations developed by professional testing agencies. In some cases, use of proficiency examinations might be a better measure of skills than written examinations. Not all certifying bodies require continuing quality of performance by persons certified, though they may require continuing membership in the association. (1974, p. 29)

Further discussion concerning the limitations of certification can be found in the *Proceedings of the 1971 Conference on Certification in Allied Health,* sponsored by the U.S. Department of Health, Education and Welfare (DHEW Publication Number NIH 73-246, September, 1971).

Accreditation A second approach that a professional organization can use for regulating the practice of an occupation is to *establish standards* for the curriculum and administration of programs that train new practitioners. Such programs may be offered by a college or university or by some other institution. (A hospital school of nursing would be an example of a professional training program that is offered by an institution other than a college or university.) By influencing the curriculums of programs that are training the practitioners for a profession, a professional organization can influence both the number of new persons who enter it and how they are trained.

A professional organization can influence the numbers of new practitioners entering a field in several ways by exercising control over curriculum. First, it can control the amount of education a person has to obtain before he or she is employable as a practitioner. The greater the amount beyond a certain level (e.g., a bachelor's degree), the fewer the number of persons who probably will be interested in entering a field, particularly if there are other fields offering similar rewards for which entrance is less costly. All else being equal, an occupation requiring a graduate degree for entrance probably would attract fewer people than one requiring a bachelor's degree.

By controlling curriculum a professional organization can influence the numbers of new practitioners entering a field in a second way: This is by limiting the numbers and sizes of training programs. It can make such programs sufficiently expensive to discourage some universities and colleges from beginning or continuing them. Or it can force training programs to limit their enrollments by establishing maximum acceptable faculty-student ratios.

By controlling curriculum a professional organization can obviously influence *how* practitioners are trained. It can influence the training not only of practitioners who will be certified as competent by it but of others as well. The American Speech-Language-Hearing Association through its accreditation program influences the training of students who will seek its certificate of clinical competence in speech-language pathology or in audiology as well as those who will not seek one of its certificates. (Such a person may seek to be licensed by a state department of education as a public school speech-language clinician.)

What is accreditation and how does it function? Accreditation is "the process by which an agency or organization evaluates or recognizes a program of study or an institution as meeting certain predetermined qualifications or standards" (Standards for federal funding, 1972, p. 547). The agency or organization is not directly (or officially) affiliated with any municipal, state, or federal governmental unit. It is likely, however, to be indirectly affiliated with one or more such units. One way by which this can occur is an agency or organization being officially recognized by a governmental unit as the regional or national accrediting body for colleges and universities as a whole or for a specific program offered by such an institution. (Colleges and universities, incidentally, are evaluated and accredited overall—as a totality—by one of six regional accrediting associations, each of which is responsible for colleges and universities located in a particular geographical region of the United States. An example of such an association would be the Middle States Association of Colleges and Schools.)

Two governmental units that can recognize accrediting organizations or agencies as "reliable authorities as to the quality of training offered by educational institutions" (Standards for federal funding, 1972, p. 547) are the National Commission on Accrediting and the U.S. Commissioner of Education. Both of these have recognized the American Speech-Language-Hearing Association as "the national accrediting agency for college and university programs offering *master's degrees* [italic mine] in speech pathology and audiology" (Standards for federal funding, 1972, p. 548). There were no organizations or agencies specifically accrediting baccalaureate or doctoral programs in these areas when this chapter was written.

A college or university training program that is accredited by an organization recognized by a national governmental unit can increase the flow of federal dollars to that program and vice versa. Accreditation by such a body has sometimes been made a requirement for eligibility to participate in funding programs sponsored by agencies of the federal government, including those providing training grants (Oulahan, 1978). The Social and Rehabilitation Services Program of the Department of Health, Education and Welfare during the early 1970s, for example, proposed to include the following in its list of criteria for determining eligibility for speech pathology and audiology training programs to participate in their training grants program:

> In order for master's degree programs to be eligible for support, they should be accredited, or be in the process of review for accreditation, by the American Speech and Hearing Association through the American Board of Examiners in Speech Pathology and Audiology and its Education and Training Board. (Standards for federal funding, 1972, p. 546)

The use of such a criterion when determining eligibility of training programs for federal support has been questioned on the basis that it tends to create a *Catch 22* situation—that is, some unaccredited programs probably could be strengthened sufficiently with federal support to achieve accreditation, but their lack of accreditation impedes their securing the federal support they need to strengthen their curriculums. Such a situation was claimed to have existed in the early 1970s for some speech-language pathology and audiology training programs in predominantly black institutions (Standards for federal funding, 1972).

The functioning of both institutional and programmatic accrediting organizations is being subjected to increasing scrutiny. Their decisions are more frequently being viewed as *judgments made by human beings* (in most cases, human beings who are attempting to function in a relatively unbiased manner) rather than as facts or truths. Partial support for this conclusion can be found in the increasing amount of litigation in which accrediting organizations are defendants (Oulahan, 1978).

Further information of a general nature about accreditation can be found in the following papers: Oulahan (1978), Roemer (1974), and *Study of Accreditation of Selected Health Education Programs—Commission Report* (1973). For additional information about accreditation of speech-language pathology and audiology master's degree training programs, see *Accreditation of Professional Education Programs in Speech Pathology and Audiology* (1977) and Standards for federal funding (1972).

Types of Regulation Administered by a Governmental Agency

There are three main ways by which a governmental agency can regulate the practice of an occupation: *individual licensure, institutional licensure,* and *registra-*

tion. The first is being used most frequently to regulate the practice of speech-language pathology and audiology as this chapter is written.

Individual Licensure Individual licensing laws are "a legal mechanism by which a governmental agency authorizes persons who have met specified minimal standards of competency to engage in a given profession or occupation" (Roemer, 1974, p. 26). Such laws can make licensure either *mandatory* or *voluntary*. If they are mandatory, they require *all* persons who practice the occupation or profession to be licensed. If, on the other hand, they are voluntary, an unlicensed person can practice, but he or she cannot claim to be licensed. Voluntary licensure, therefore, can be viewed as a form of *governmental certification* (Roemer, 1974). Most licensure laws that regulate the practice of speech-language pathology and audiology are of the mandatory type.

Occupational licensing is almost always a responsibility of *state* rather than federal or municipal government. As a result, the requirements for being licensed to practice a given occupation are apt to differ from state to state. While such differences in requirements for licensure are minimal for some occupations, they are substantial for others. As this chapter is written, some states require a master's degree to be licensed as a public school speech-language pathologist and others require only a bachelor's degree.

The standards under which an occupation is licensed in a particular state are specified in a statute enacted by the legislature of that state. This statute, among other things, establishes a licensing board for that occupation. This board, which functions as an administrative agency (see Chapter 2), has the responsibility for implementing the licensure program mandated by the statute. Its members may or may not *all* be practitioners of the occupation. Those who are not are likely to represent consumers of its services. (Occupations usually seek to limit membership on this board to their practitioners.) The board is almost always required by the state to be self-supporting, with expenses met by licensing fees. Such fees for a particular occupation can vary considerably from state to state. Their magnitude, in part, would be a function of the number of persons residing in a state who are likely to seek licensure for that occupation—the larger the number of such persons, the lower the fees are apt to be (Governmental regulation, 1969).

The formulation and passage of a state occupational licensing law (particularly one that is mandatory) is likely to cost the practitioners of the occupation (through their state association) a great deal, in terms of both time and money. They may have to retain a lobbyist to guide their bill through the legislative process, and they have no guarantee that the lobbyist's efforts will be successful. If they are successful, practitioners will have to pay a license fee. Considering the financial and time investments involved, why would they seek to have their occupation licensed? Several possible reasons are suggested in the following paragraphs.

The primary justification for licensure is the protection of the public. Protection of the public has broader implications than physical damage or loss of life. Unless it can be shown that the public needs protection, attempts to secure licensing regulations are not likely to succeed. . . .

In addition to the primary justification mentioned above, there are other important reasons for desiring legislation. For example, licensure of a profession is perhaps the most stringent defense against encroachment on its activities from another profession. . . . Further, licensing legislation tends to force rigorous definition of the activity involved. Finally, the economic advantages of licensure to the licensed group have been clearly recognized. (Governmental regulation, 1969, p. 41)

The fact that the practitioners of an occupation have succeeded in having a state legislature pass a licensure law does not necessarily mean that their involvement with that legislature has ended. They may have to ask it at some future time to change the requirements for licensure so that these requirements are consistent with how practitioners are being trained. They also may have to convince it to not allow their licensure program to terminate. Some states have sunset laws under which administrative agencies (such as occupational licensing boards) are terminated at the end of a specified number of years unless the legislature acts to retain them. A legislature is unlikely to act to retain an agency unless it can be convinced that the agency is performing an essential function. Obviously, if an occupational licensing board is scheduled to be terminated and the practitioners of that occupation wish it to be retained, they are going to have to convince the members of the legislature that it performs an important function. (For further information concerning sunset laws and occupational licensing, see Downey 1979.)

A number of states have passed or are seeking to pass licensing laws for speech-language pathologists and audiologists. These laws are summarized in a publication of the American Speech-Language-Hearing Association titled *State Legislation.*

Institutional Licensure Institutional licensure has existed for more than twenty-five years. Until recently it has been concerned almost exclusively with the quality of facilities (e.g., sanitation and fire safety). Under this form of licensure certain aspects of the functioning of an institution (e.g., a hospital or rehabilitation center) are monitored by a government agency; so long as the institution conforms to certain minimum standards, it remains licensed to perform its function. The government agency would tend to be concerned primarily about whether its standards were being met rather than the means by which the institution was meeting them. So long as the institution meets them by lawful means, the agency is unlikely to interfere.

There have been attempts since the early 1970s to extend institutional licensure to include regulating the quality of services provided by an institution (Levine, 1978). Although these attempts for the most part have been unsuccessful, they may foreshadow a movement that at some future time could have a significant impact on the practice of speech-language pathology and audiology. Such a movement could have a profound impact on the practice of these professions because the agency monitoring a hospital, rehabilitation center, nursing home, or other institution providing clinical speech, language, and/or hearing services is likely to have as its focus the quality of the services provided—that is, whether the services meet *minimum* standards with regard to quality. If the speech, language, and hearing services provided by an institution met the agency's minimum standards, it may not be concerned about whether the persons providing them are licensed by the state or certified by their professional association (particularly the latter). The institution, in a sense, would assume the responsiblity for establishing qualifications for persons providing the various services that it offers. Such qualifications *may* or *may not* conform to those for individual licensure or certification.

Institutional licensure, if it were adopted, could have a significant impact on the practice of speech-language pathology and audiology in such institutions as hospitals, rehabilitation centers, and nursing homes. A hospital, for example, could hire a person who has a bachelor's degree with a major in speech-language pathology or audiology to do basic hearing testing. So long as the hospital could demonstrate that the person was capable of doing such hearing testing with results that possessed at least a minimally acceptable level of validity and reliability and that the person would refer cases requiring more sophisticated testing than he or she could provide, the government agency monitoring the institution would be unlikely to be concerned about the fact that the services were being provided by someone who was neither licensed nor certified in audiology. In fact, it is conceivable that the institution could be commended for not using an expensive, "overqualified" person to provide these services.

Most organizations representing health-related professionals are opposed to that aspect of institutional licensure concerned with establishing qualifications for personnel (Levine, 1978). They fear that some institutions, to reduce costs, might be tempted to hire practitioners who lack the qualifications for securing the appropriate state licensure or professional certification. They also have reservations about the ability of those doing the hiring at institutions (who may not be practitioners in their field) to establish qualifications for serving as practitioners in their field if they choose not to use the qualifications for the existing state license or professional certificate. Because of the less than enthusiastic reception that the concept of institutional licensure of personnel has received in many professional circles, it is doubtful that it will replace individual licensure or certification in the immediate future. It is likely, however, to *coexist* with them in a limited form. (This is already occurring in some institutions with regard to the paraprofessional speech clinician designated as a *communication aid*. The qualifications for persons functioning in this capacity are currently being established by the institutions employing them.)

Registration Registration is a form of certification that is administered by a governmental agency. Persons who have completed the training deemed necessary by the agency to function as a practitioner in a particular field have their names listed in a register (file) that is maintained by that agency. A person may be able to become registered by graduating from a training program that is accredited by the agency.

The certificates that speech-language pathologists obtain from state departments of public instruction that allow them to work in public schools can be viewed as a form of registration. Speech-language pathologists can be registered almost automatically by completing a training program that is accredited by their state department of education.

WHAT APPROACHES HAVE BEEN USED TO REGULATE THE PRACTICE OF SPEECH-LANGUAGE PATHOLOGY AND AUDIOLOGY?

Thus far in this chapter we have explored both the motivation for regulating the practice of an occupation and the approaches that can be used for this purpose. This section deals with the manner in which these approaches have been used for regulating the practice of speech-language pathology and audiology. The information presented is quite general because the requirements for certification, licensure, accreditation, and registration have been and are likely to continue to be revised frequently.

Certification

The professional association that is most actively involved in the clinical certification of speech-language pathologists and audiologists is the American Speech-Language-Hearing Association (ASHA). ASHA has been certifying the clinical competence of practitioners in communicative disorders since the early 1950s. It currently offers two certificates of clinical competence—one in speech-language pathology and one in audiology. Both require an applicant to have earned a masters degree, to have completed a prescribed program of academic and clinical practicum experiences, to have completed a clinical fellowship year (i.e., an internship), to have agreed to conform to a code of ethics, and to have passed a national examination. Write to the American Speech-Language-Hearing Association for specific information concerning the requirements for these certificates and others they may be offering.

ASHA is not the only association that offers certification relevant to the practice of speech-language pathology and audiology. A number of professional associations and groups offer *speciality certification* that would be of interest to some speech-language pathologists and audiologists. Almost all of these speciality certificates are for either the administration and interpretation of a diagnostic test, such as the *Porch Index of Communicative Ability* (Porch, 1967), or the application of a therapy approach, such as Blissymbolics (Kates, McNaughton, and Silverman, no date).

Accreditation

The American Speech-Language-Hearing Association maintains a voluntary accreditation program for master's degree training programs in speech-language pathology and audiology. Both a listing of accredited programs and specific information about requirements for accreditation can be obtained from ASHA.

Licensure

A number of states require speech-language pathologists and audiologists who are not employed by public schools to be licensed. To find out whether a state in which you plan to practice has such a requirement, contact that state's speech and hearing association. The specific requirements for licensure (if a state requires it) can be obtained from the state agency (board) responsible for administering the program.

The American Speech-Language-Hearing Association, in its publication *State Legislation,* includes summaries of licensing laws for speech-language pathologists and audiologists and for hearing aid dealers. ASHA also publishes the periodical *Governmental Affairs Review,* which includes information on state licensure.

Registration

The certification that a speech-language pathologist must obtain to be employable in the public schools of a particular state can be viewed as a form of registration. (The rationale for viewing it in this manner is presented elsewhere in this chapter.) The requirements for such certification vary widely from state to state. Those for a particular state can be obtained from its department of public instruction.

HOW CAN CERTIFICATION, ACCREDITATION, LICENSURE, OR REGISTRATION BE LOST?

When individuals have achieved certification, licensure, or registration or when training programs have been accredited, it is tempting for the individuals or institutions to assume that their new status is permanent. This is not necessarily true! Certification, licensure, registration, and accreditation can be lost for a variety of reasons. Some of the more common reasons are described in this section.

Reasons for Loss of Certification, Licensure, and Registration

Failure to Abide by the Code of Ethics   A requirement for almost any form of occupational certification, licensure, or registration is agreeing to be *ethical* in one's interactions with consumers and fellow professionals. Unfortunately, the categorization of behavior as ethical or unethical involves a *value judgment*—there probably is no behavior that would be categorized as either ethical or unethical by most persons under *all* circumstances. This being the case, how does a governmental agency or a professional association determine whether particular behavior is unethical? They usually do this by operationally defining (Bridgman, 1961) behaving ethically as adhering to a code of ethics. The code of ethics consists of a set of behaviors that can occur in interactions between practitioners and consumers and between practitioners and other professionals, some of which are regarded as ethical and others as unethical. If a practitioner does something that is *prohibited* by the code of ethics or fails to so something that the code *requires,* he or she can be classified as behaving in an unethical manner and can lose his license, certification, or registration. For further information about codes of professional ethics see Chapter 5.

Failure to Maintain Membership in the Certifying Organization or to Pay Required Fees Some certifying organizations (including the American Speech-Language-Hearing Association) require persons to whom they have awarded certification to either maintain membership in them or to pay an annual fee, which is regarded as their fair share of the costs to the organization of maintaining the certification program. Failure to maintain membership in the organization or to pay the annual fee can result in loss of certification. Also, failure to pay annual licensing and registration fees (if there are any) can result in loss of these credentials.

Failure to Comply with Changes in Requirements for the Certification, Licensure, or Registration The requirements for a given type of certification, licensure, or registration are likely to change from time to time. Are persons who are already certified, licensed, or registered required to meet new requirements? The answer to this question depends on whether there is a grandfather clause and, if there is, what it covers. A grandfather clause excuses a person who is already certified, licensed, or registered from having to meet some new requirements, but not necessarily all new requirements. For example, such a clause is unlikely to excuse one from a new requirement for participation in continuing education.

The Certification, Licensure, or Registration Being Terminated A person may lose one of these credentials because the program under which it was awarded is terminated. Of the three, a speech-language pathologist or audiologist is most likely to lose licensure in this manner. A number of states have enacted sunset laws (Downey, 1979) that affect their licensure boards. When such a law has been enacted, a licensure board is automatically terminated after a certain number of years unless the legislature votes to continue it.

Reasons for Loss of Accreditation

A training program can lose its accreditation for several reasons, singly or in combination. First, it can be judged to no longer be meeting the standards under which it was accredited. This can happen if faculty leave and are not replaced by persons who, in the judgment of the accrediting agency, are competent to teach their courses. Second, the program can be judged as unable to meet the standards in effect when it is considered for reaccreditation. The accreditation awarded by most organizations, including the American Speech-Language-Hearing Association, is for a finite number of years. If a training program wishes to remain accredited, it must apply for reaccreditation at the end of this period. And third, it may choose not to apply for reaccreditation when its accreditation terminates. For example, a training program may choose not to apply for reaccreditation because the faculty believes that the program does not meet current standards for accreditation.

PROCEDURES USED FOR TAKING AWAY CERTIFICATION, ACCREDITATION, LICENSURE, AND REGISTRATION

The procedures that are used by a professional association or governmental agency for taking away the license, registration, or certification of a practitioner or the accreditation of a training program are *supposed* to be consistent with the concept of *due process* (specifically, procedural due process), which can be viewed as one of the cornerstones of our legal system. If due process is being adhered to in such procedures, the person or training program in question will be informed of the charges that have been made and will be given an opportunity to answer them. This can involve a hearing during which the agency or association and the individual or training program present evidence to a hearing officer supporting their contentions that the credential should and should not be taken away. Both parties are likely to be represented by attorneys. Following presentation of the evidence, the hearing officer (who is supposed to be unbiased) decides whether the *preponderance of evidence* supports the charges made by the agency or association. If in his or her judgment the preponderance of evidence supports the charges that were made, the hearing officer *can* order that the licensure, registration, certification, or accreditation be taken away. (Of course, a hearing officer probably would not order revocation if he or she felt that the charges, though proven, were not serious enough to warrant such action.) On the other hand, if the hearing officers feels that the preponderance of evidence does not support these charges, he or she is supposed to order the agency or association not to take away the credential.

If the person or training program involved feels that the decision of the hearing officer was not warranted by the evidence that was presented, the person or program should have the right to *appeal* it. At least one level of appeal within the agency or association will be possible in most cases. If the person or training program remains dissatisfied with the decision after exhausting all possibilities for appeal within the association or agency, he, or she, or the program can initiate a *civil suit* against the agency or association in an appropriate state or federal court. The procedures by which such a suit would be initiated and conducted are outlined in Chapter 2.

In some cases the charges made can be answered without the need for a formal hearing. The association or agency can present the person or program with a written statement of the charges and ask that he, she, or the program *show cause* (in writing) why the credential should not be taken away. If the charges lack merit, it may be possible to resolve the situation in this manner. The American Speech-Language-Hearing Association has used this approach in its clinical certification and accreditation programs.

Write to the American Speech-Language-Hearing Association for specific information about appeals procedures in its clinical certification and accreditation programs. For comparable information about state licensure and registration programs contact the appropriate agency (e.g., state licensing board or department of public instruction).

REFERENCES

Accreditation of Professional Education Programs in Speech Pathology and Audiology. Rockville, Md.: American Speech-Language-Hearing Association (1977).
BRIDGMAN, P. W., *The Logic of Modern Physics.* New York: Macmillan (1961).
DOWNEY, M., Legal developments—Antitrust and sunset laws. *Asha,* 21, 7-11 (1979).
Governmental regulation: A statement by the American Speech and Hearing Association. *Asha,* 11, 39-43 (1969).
KATES, B., MCNAUGHTON, S., and SILVERMAN, H., *Handbook of Blissymbolics for Instructors, Users, Parents and Administrators.* Toronto: Blissymbolics Communication Institute (no date).
KATZ, J., BASIL, R. A., and SMITH, J. M., A staggered spondaic test for detecting central auditory lesions. *Annals of Otology, Rhinology, and Laryngology,* 72, 908-918 (1963).
LEVINE, L. B., Institutional licensure versus individual licensure. *Journal of Allied Health,* 7, 109-114 (1978).
LUM, J., Reference groups and professional socialization. In Margaret Hardy and Mary E. Conway (Eds.), *Role Theory: Prospectives for Health Professionals.* Englewood Cliffs, N.J.: Prentice-Hall (1979).
OULAHAN, C., The legal implications of evaluation and accreditation. *Journal of Law and Education,* 7, 193-238 (1978).
PORCH, B. E., *Porch Index of Communicative Ability.* Palo Alto, Calif.: Consulting Psychologists Press (1967).
Position statement on nonspeech communication. *Asha,* 23, 577-581 (1981).
ROEMER, R., Trends in licensure, certification, and accreditation: Implications for health-manpower education in the future. *Journal of Allied Health,* 3, 26-33 (1974).
ROTTENBERG, S., Licensing, occupational. In D. L. Sills (Ed.), *International Encyclopedia of the Social Sciences.* Volume 9. New York: Macmillan and Free Press, 283-285 (1968).
Standards for federal funding. *Asha,* 14, 546-550 (1972).
Study of Accreditation of Selected Health Education Programs—Commission Report. Washington, D.C.: Department of Health, Education and Welfare (1973).
WEBSTER, R. A., A behavioral analysis of stuttering: Treatment and theory. In K. Calhoun et al. (Eds.), *Innovative Treatment Methods in Psychopathology.* New York: John Wiley (1974).

4

Contractual Obligations to Clients and Others

In our society it is almost impossible to be completely self-sufficient. We rely on others to provide almost all of the goods and services we consume. This mandatory reliance on others has several implications. First, it means we need a mechanism to ensure that a person who agrees to provide us with certain goods and services does what he or she *promises*. And second, it means we need a mechanism for ensuring that a person who provides goods and services for another will be fairly compensated for them (usually by being given money). The legal mechanism used in our society to enforce promises is the *contract*. Without a mechanism for enforcing promises, a society such as ours in which we must rely on others to satisfy most of our needs would be impossible.

We are constantly entering into contracts in both our personal and professional lives. We are usually not consciously aware of doing so because we tend to view contracts as written documents that must be signed to be enforceable. A contract does *not* have to be written to be enforceable. Under certain circumstances *oral promises* (both direct and implied) are enforceable as contracts. And even *written documents* that are labeled contracts are *not* enforceable as contracts under certain circumstances. Thus, some promises that appear to be enforceable as contracts are not and others that do not appear to be enforceable as contracts are enforceable as contracts. Since we cannot avoid entering into contracts, we must be able to recognize when we are doing so and what the implications are. My overall objective in this chapter is to increase your level of awareness and understanding of the contracts you enter into, particularly those you enter into when functioning professionally as a speech-language pathologist or audiologist.

EVENTS THAT CAN RESULT IN THE CREATION OF A CONTRACT

A contract is an *enforceable promise*. It is described in the authoritative work, *Restatement of the Law: Contracts,* in the following manner: "A contract is a promise for the breach of which the law gives a remedy, or the performance of which the law in some way recognizes as a duty" (1973, p. 5). Thus a contract is a promise (or a set of promises) that a court is likely to enforce if it is asked to do so. The qualifier "is likely" was used here because the courts do not always do what they would be expected to do. Also, the phrase "if it is asked to do so" was added because a court cannot become involved in the enforcement of a contract unless the person to whom the promise that was not kept was made initiates a *civil suit* (see Chapter 2 for a discussion of civil suits). The threat of such a suit, incidentally, may be enough to motivate a person to do what he or she promised, for being a defendant in a suit that is likely to be successful can result in expensive attorney's fees and court costs.

Contracts also have been defined as *enforceable agreements.* When people enter into a contractual relationship they usually agree to do certain things for each other. For example, an audiologist agrees to test a child's hearing, and the parents *agree* to pay him or her a certain amount of money for performing this service. The word *agreement* is sometimes used in written contracts in place of the word *contract.*

What role does contract law play in our legal system? As we saw in Chapter 2 the laws that make up our legal system impose *restrictions and obligations* on our behavior. These restrictions and obligations are of two types: *involuntary* and *voluntary.* We are required to behave in a manner consistent with the first type, which are the majority, *regardless of whether we have explicitly promised or agreed to do so.* (We indirectly promise or agree to obey such laws by residing in our country and thereby in our state and municipality.) The sources of such laws include federal, state, and municipal legislatures; adminstrative agencies; and court decisions (i.e., common law).

The second type of law that imposes restrictions and obligations on our behavior we voluntarily agree to obey. These laws are created by *private individuals* rather than legislatures, government agencies, or court decisions. They are private rather than public laws. They impose restrictions and obligations on the behavior of only a relatively small number of persons—often as few as two. They do not duplicate public laws but supplement them. Thus, contract law provides a mechanism for imposing restrictions and obligations on behavior in some situations— interactions between people—that are not regulated by public law.

Though contracts are private laws, they are enforced by the *courts,* the same institution that enforces public laws. The courts, through their common lawmaking function, have established rules for *creating* and *enforcing* contracts. A contract that is created in a manner consistent with these rules will be enforced by the courts. Hence, it is necessary to understand these rules in order to understand how certain events can result in the creation of a contract. My objective in this section is to help you to develop an intuitive understanding of some of the more basic of these rules, including those pertaining to (1) the *offer,* or promise, (2) the *acceptance* of the offer, and (3) the *consideration* exchanged by the parties, or what they voluntarily agree to relinquish or do for each other that is supposed to motivate them to keep the promises they made in the contract.

The Offer (Promise)

The first event that must occur for a contract to be created is the act of *making an offer.* A speech-language pathologist, for example, can offer to include an adult stutterer in an ongoing group therapy program. The person who makes the offer is referred to as the *offeror* and the person to whom it is made is referred to as the *offeree.* Thus, the speech-language pathologist in this example would be the offeror and the adult stutterer would be the offeree.

The offer-making process almost always involves the offeror conveying to the offeree (1) what he or she will do for the offeree and (2) what he or she expects in return from the offeree. The word *conveying* was used here rather than *saying* and/or *writing* because an offer can be conveyed without the use of spoken or written language. It can be conveyed by implication. Thus, "A promise may be stated in words either oral or written, or may be inferred wholly or partially from conduct" (*Restatement of the Law: Contracts,* 1973, p. 12). The following is an example of a situation in which an offer is conveyed without words:

> A, on passing a market, where he has an account, sees a box of apples marked "5 cts. each." A picks up an apple, holds it up so that a clerk of the establishment sees the act. The clerk nods, and A passes on. A has promised to pay five cents for the apple. (*Restatement of the Law: Contracts,* 1973, pp. 12-13)

Similarly, a hard-of-hearing adult who seeks and accepts a hearing aid evaluation from an audiologist conveys to that audiologist by implication a promise to pay him (or have a third party pay him) a reasonable fee for the evaluation. (The presumption in our society is that people are willing to pay a reasonable fee for professional services that they ask for and receive.)

Theoretically, it should be a relatively easy task to determine whether an offer has been made. All one should have to establish is whether a promise was conveyed from offeror to offeree by words, or by implication, or by some combination of the two. Unfortunately, this may *not* be an easy task. It depends on what an objective observer (i.e., a "reasonable person") would have perceived to be the *intent* of the offeror when he or she said, or wrote, or did that which could be construed as an offer. According to Fisher:

> Whether an offer has been made depends on *intent*—the objective intent of a reasonable man observing the actions claimed to constitute the offer. It is not the subjective intent of the offeror that controls the determination of whether an offer has been made. (1977, p. 418)

Thus when attempting to determine whether an offer had been made a judge would consider if a *reasonable person* hearing or seeing the words or observing the actions that are claimed to convey the offer would conclude that an offer had been made. If the judge feels that a reasonable person would have been likely to perceive those words and/or actions as conveying an offer, he or she would probably rule that the intent was to make an offer. On the other hand, if the judge feels that a *reasonable person* would have been *unlikely* to perceive those words and/or actions as conveying an offer, he or she probably will rule that they do not constitute an offer. Since there probably will be no way for the judge to establish the *subjective* intent of the offeror, the judge, one would hope, will not include what he or she thinks the intent was as a factor in the decision (i.e., ruling).

It is desirable that offers be as specific, or unambiguous, as possible. The more specific an offer, the more likely both offeror and offeree will agree on what is being proposed, that is, the obligations they will be expected to assume if the offer is accepted. Also, if the offer is accepted and becomes a contract, a court will have less difficulty determining whether the contract has been breached (violated) if the language is relatively specific, or unambiguous. In this regard, it is particularly important that when a speech-language pathologist or audiologist offers clinical services to a communicatively handicapped person, the person and/or the family understands that the offer does not promise *(guarantee)* a cure or a specific level of improvement. All that can be promised (guaranteed) is that the speech-language pathologist or audiologist will make a *reasonable attempt* to assist the person in reducing the severity of the communicative disorder for as long a period as it is reasonable to expect significant further improvement to be possible. A judge would be unlikely to view the failure of speech-language pathology or audiology services to significantly reduce the severity of a person's communicative disorder to constitute a *breach of contract* if a reasonable attempt was made to assist the person in reducing the severity of the communicative disorder and if improvement could reasonably be expected. However, a judge would be likely to view this as constituting a breach of contract if clinical services were being provided when there was no reasonable hope for significant improvement (unless the person or family, after being informed that the prognosis for further improvement was extremely poor, requested *in writing* that therapy services be continued). Providing a client with clinical services when there is no reasonable hope for improvement could also be viewed as a violation of the American Speech-Language-Hearing Association Code of Ethics (see Chapter 5 for a discussion of professional ethics).

An offer must be *formally communicated* before it can be accepted and become a contract. What constitutes formal communication is the use of a *medium* (such as a letter) that is normally used for communicating such offers. If you heard "through the grapevine" that you had been awarded a grant for which you had applied, you ordinarily could not sue the organization awarding it for breach of contract if they changed their mind before formally communicating (probably in writing) to you an offer of the award.

An offeror usually can withdraw, or terminate, an offer during the period between when it is communicated to the offeree and the offeree formally accepts it. There are a variety of reasons an offeror might do this. One is particularly relevant to clinical practice—that is, *lapse of a reasonable time.* A person who is offered clinical services by a speech-language pathologist or audiologist should be given a reasonable period of time to decide whether to accept them. When the services are offered, the prospective client should be told how much time he or she has to accept the offer. If the client does not accept within this time period, the clinician is no longer obliged to either reserve a slot in the schedule for the person or to provide the services offered for the agreed fee.

Acceptance of the Offer

The second event that must occur for a contract to be formed is the *acceptance* of the offer by the offeree. An adult stutterer, for example, may accept a speech-language pathologist's offer to enroll her in a therapy group.

If an offeree wishes to accept an offer and thereby establish a contract, how should he or she do it? "Acceptance of an offer is a manifestation of assent to the terms thereof made by the offeree in a manner invited or required by the offer" (*Restatement of the Law: Contracts,* 1973, p. 108). Thus, an offeree can accept an offer—that is, the *totality* of what has been offered—by indicating a desire to do so in the manner specified by the offeror (e.g., by signing a contract). If the offeror does not specify how acceptance should be manifested, then any reasonable mode can be used.

There are two basic ways by which acceptance of an offer can be manifested, or indicated. The first of these is acceptance by *performance.* "Acceptance by performance requires that at least part of what the offer requests be performed or tendered and includes acceptance by a performance which operates as a return promise" (*Restatement of the Law: Contracts,* 1973, p. 108). Thus, an offeree can indicate acceptance *without words* by beginning to do what acceptance of the offer would require him or her to do, assuming the offer has not been withdrawn or terminated. An adult stutterer could accept a speech-language pathologist's offer of enrollment in a particular ongoing therapy group by attending one or more sessions of that group. Or an audiologist could accept an offer to screen the hearing of the children enrolled in a private school by beginning to screen their hearing.

The second way acceptance can be manifested is by a *promise.* "Acceptance by a promise requires that the offeree complete every act essential to the making of the promise" (*Restatement of the Law: Contracts,* 1973, p. 108). In this case, an offeree would accept an offer by *promising* to do what is required by the offer. He or she may make the promise in words or other symbols (e.g., manual signs) or may imply the promise by conduct. A speech-language pathologist or audiologist in private practice would be accepting an offer by making a promise when he or she signed a *lease* for an office (the lease being a contract). The promise includes the payment of a certain amount of money to the offeror for rent each month for the duration of the lease.

The courts ordinarily do not interpret an offeree's *silence* (i.e., failure to notify the offeror that he or she does not wish to accept the offer) as conveying acceptance. Thus, if a speech-language pathologist told an adult stutterer that he will assume the stutterer wishes to be enrolled in the therapy group unless he is informed to the contrary before the end of the month, he would be on shaky ground. The courts ordinarily will rule that an offer has not been accepted unless the offeree conveys acceptance by performance or by making a promise. One of the few exceptions that speech-language pathologists and audiologists are likely to encounter is related to delivery of the main selection in book clubs. Most of these clubs will ship the main selection *offered* each month to you if you *fail to notify* them within a specified period of time that you don't want it. Here silence after being offered the main selection is interpreted as indicating acceptance of the offer because you agreed to this when you joined.

The offeree must accept the offer in its *entirety* for a contract to be formed. He or she cannot accept only parts of it. If an offeree is willing to accept parts of it, he or she can convey to the offeror a statement of the parts he or she is willing to accept. This statement would be regarded as a *counteroffer*. The making of a counteroffer terminates the offeror's original offer.

The Consideration Exchanged by the Parties

Acceptance of an offer will only result in the formation of a contract *if certain conditions are met.* (An in-depth discussion of these conditions is presented in the volumes *Corbin on Contracts*, 1952, and *Restatement of the Law: Contracts*, 1973.) One of the most important is that *consideration* be exchanged by the parties. "Consideration embraces the idea that there should be a voluntary relinquishment of a known right by the respective parties to one another for there to be an enforceable agreement by either of them against the other" (Fisher, 1977, p. 449). The courts tend to view it as only fair that *both* offeror and offeree voluntarily agree to give up something (i.e., to assume an obligation that would not have to be assumed if there were no contract). The courts ordinarily will not enforce a contract in which one or both parties failed to voluntarily relinquish a known right.

What constitutes consideration perhaps can be made clearer by describing the two forms it can take. The *first* is that the offeree in accepting an offer agrees to give up something that belongs to the offeree that could *benefit* the offeror. For example, a hard-of-hearing person (offeror) offers to buy a hearing aid from an audiologist (offeree) for $500. The audiologist accepts the offer and delivers the hearing aid to the hard-of-hearing person. The transfer and delivery of the hearing aid constitutes consideration because in exchange for a promise to pay him $500 the audiologist has voluntarily relinquished something that he owns (i.e., a hearing aid) that should *benefit* the hard-of-hearing person. The hard-of-hearing person, in turn, would be voluntarily relinquishing something that belongs to him—$500.

The *second form* that consideration can take is that the offeree in accepting an offer agrees to do something that would be recognized by the courts as having a *detrimental* effect on him or her (i.e., cause the offeree to do something he or she wouldn't choose to do) rather than having a beneficial effect on the offeror. The following example illustrates this form of consideration:

> A promises B, his nephew aged 16, that A will pay B $1000 when B becomes 21 if B does not smoke before then. B's forebearance to smoke is a performance and if bargained for is consideration for A's promise. (*Restatement of the Law: Contracts,* 1973, p. 152)

The phrase *bargained for,* as used here, implies that the money offered was not merely a gift. The assumption is being made that B would have smoked if his uncle hadn't made the offer. Thus, in not smoking he would voluntarily be relinquishing a right. It, of course, could be argued that the uncle was receiving a psychological benefit—that is, not having to cope with a nephew who smokes.

For an act to constitute consideration, what is being relinquished by performing the act must be an *actual* (real) known right. Agreeing to do for someone something that one is required to do by law ordinarily would not constitute consideration. Since we are expected to meet our legal obligations, then doing something we are obliged to do anyway would not constitute relinquishing a known right. Thus, in the following example there is no act that is likely to be construed by a court as constituting consideration since a police officer has a legal duty to produce evidence.

> A offers a reward to whoever produces evidence leading to the arrest and conviction of the murderer of B. C produces such evidence in the performance of his duty as a police officer. C's performance is not consideration for A's promise. (*Restatement of the Law: Contracts,* 1973, p. 157)

If a public school speech-language pathologist made an offer to the parents of a communicatively handicapped child to include their child in her caseload in exchange for a payment of $100 and they accepted, the clinician probably would be unsuccessful in suing the parents for breach of contract if they did not pay her $100 after she included the child in the caseload. The clinician was not relinquishing a right by offering to provide clinical services for the child because her contract with the local school district required her to provide such services.

Events That Can Interfere with the Creation of an Enforceable Contract

There are several categories of events other than a problem with consideration that can lead to the acceptance of an offer not resulting in an enforceable contract.

They will be dealt with briefly in this section. (For additional information see Corbin, 1952, Fisher, 1977, and *Restatement of the Law: Contracts,* 1973.)

The reasons why acceptance of an offer may not result in an enforceable contract include the following: (1) incapacity, (2) fraud, (3) mistake, (4) duress, (5) the offer being unconscionable, (6) illegality, and (7) the contract not being in written form when it was required to be. A court may legally excuse a party to a "contract" from meeting his or her contractual obligations if it can be established that *there is no contract* because of one or more of these reasons. For the acceptance of an offer to result in the creation of a contract the *assumption* has to be made that the parties have the mental and legal *capacity* to enter into a contract, that one party is not attempting to commit a *fraud* on the other, that the contract actually was accepted and reflects the agreement (i.e., it contains no *mistakes* that can influence its interpretation), that the offeree did not accept the offer under *duress,* and so forth. A court is likely to rule that no contract exists and, hence, neither party can seek damages for its being breached if it can be demonstrated that this assumption is not viable. These reasons why acceptance of an offer may not result in an enforceable contract are of more than academic interest. *They can provide a legal means for escaping from the obligations that you are required by a contract to assume. They also can result in the courts' nullifying a contract in which you are the offeror.*

Incapacity The law requires that a person who is accepting an offer have the *mental capacity* to understand the obligations he or she is assuming for the acceptance to result in the formation of a contract. If it can be established that a person lacks such mental capacity, a court is likely to rule that any contracts he or she enters into are unenforceable.

Several categories of persons are almost always assumed by the courts to lack the mental capacity needed to knowledgeably enter into at least some contractual relationships. These include persons who have not as yet reached the *age of majority* (children) and persons who are intoxicated. Also included are persons who have been diagnosed as *mentally ill* or *mentally defective.*

A person can usually escape from having to meet at least some contractual obligations by reason of mental incapacity if one or both of the following can be established:

(a) he is unable to understand in a reasonable manner the nature and consequences of the transaction, or
(b) he is unable to act in a reasonable manner in relation to the transaction and the other party has reason to know of his condition. (*Restatement of the Law: Contracts,* 1973, p. 33)

One or both probably could be established for persons diagnosed as moderately or severely *mentally retarded* or for those diagnosed as *senile.* It may also be possible to establish one or both for persons who have certain *communicative disorders* resulting from damage to the central nervous system. It could be argued, for example, that a person who had receptive aphasia who accepted an offer was "unable to understand in a reasonable manner the nature and consequences of the transaction." A speech-language pathologist, incidentally, might be asked to testify whether in his or her *professional opinion* it is likely that a receptive aphasic who entered into a contract was able "to understand in a reasonable manner the nature and consequences of the transaction." (See Chapter 11 for a discussion of the role of the speech-language pathologist and audiologist as an *expert witness.)*

Mental incapacity as defined by these two criteria is of concern to audiologists as well as speech-language pathologists. It could be argued, for example, that a *deaf* person who accepted an offer was "unable to understand in a reasonable manner the nature and consequences of the transaction." For an in-depth discussion of the implications of the offeree's being deaf on the acceptance of an offer (and, hence, on the creation of a contract), see Section 12 in Meyers, *The Law and the Deaf* (1968).

The courts may be unwilling to allow someone to escape from meeting all contractual obligations because of mental incapacity. They may rule that a person is mentally competent to enter into some contractual relationships but not into others. Also, a person may be unable to avoid meeting contractual obligations because the offeror was unaware of his or her mental condition. Some of the issues involved in determining competency are summarized in the following paragraph from the authoritative work, *Restatement of the Law: Contracts:*

> *The standard of competency.* It is now recognized that there is a wide variety of types and degrees of mental incompetency. Among them are congenital deficiencies in intelligence, the mental deterioration of old age, *the effects of brain damage caused by accident or organic disease* [italics mine], and mental illness evidenced by such symptoms as delusions, hallucinations, delirium, confusion and depression. Where a guardian has been appointed [by a court], there is full contractual capacity in any case unless the mental illness or defect has affected the particular transaction: a person may be able to understand almost nothing, or only simple or routine transactions, or he may be incompetent only with respect to a particular type of transaction. Even though understanding is complete, he may lack capacity to control his acts in the way that the normal individual can and does control them; in such cases the incapacity makes the contract voidable only if the other party has reason to know of his condition. Where a person has some understanding of a particular transaction which is affected by mental illness or defect, the controlling consideration is whether the transaction in its result is one which a reasonably competent person might have made. (1973, p. 34)

Fraud Fraud is "an intentional perversion of truth for the purpose of inducing another in reliance upon it to part with some valuable thing belonging to him or to surrender a legal right . . ." (Black, 1968, p. 788). An offeror committing a fraud would *intentionally* provide false information to the offeree to induce acceptance of an offer. The offeror by behaving in this manner is attempting to *defraud* the offeree.

A person who has been defrauded has several options. He or she can ask a court for a release from the contractual obligations—that is, ask for the court to rule that no contract exists. Or the person can force the offeror to live up to the contractual obligations if he or she feels that this would be advantageous to him or her (or disadvantageous to the offeror). A contractual relationship that a person was induced to enter because of fraud may become one from which he or she can derive some benefit due to a *change in circumstances.* Suppose, for example, an audiologist agrees to screen the employees at a factory at some future time for $1000 after the company *intentionally* leads her to believe that the factory employs fewer people than it does. When the time comes for her to do the screening, she is informed that a significant percentage of the employees have been laid off. Thus, because of a change in circumstances (i.e., fewer employees to screen) the fee she was promised might be more than adequate to compensate her for doing the screening. A court would be unlikely to release the company from its contractual obligation if asked to do so because it originally intended to defraud the audiologist. A judge, in fact, is apt to view enforcement of the contract as yielding poetic justice!

Mistake A mistake is an *"unintentional* [italics mine] act, omission, or error arising from ignorance, surprise, ... or misplaced confidence" (Black, 1968, p. 1152). A mistake can be made by either the offeror or offeree that results in a contract which one or both parties view as unfair.

Our concern here is the impact "of action that has been induced by a mistaken thought" (Corbin, 1952, p. 539) on the enforceability of contracts. An offeree may accept an offer *(action)* because he or she misunderstood (was *mistaken* about) what was being offered. Or an offeror may *act* on the belief that the offeree has accepted the offer when the offeree did not intend to do so. The offeror's action in such an instance would have been "induced by a mistaken thought." (This type of mistake, incidentally, can be prevented by having a *written* contract: The offeree by signing the contract indicates unequivocally that he or she wishes to accept the offer.) Or a person may make an offer *in jest* that is accepted on the mistaken belief that it was a serious offer. Or an offeree may accept an offer (e.g., sign a contract) on the mistaken belief that the information presented in it is accurate, but the offeror *unintentionally* included inaccurate information in it. In all of these situations the *possibility* exists of a court's ruling that no contract exists because acceptance of the offer did not involve a true "meeting of minds." However, there is no guarantee that a court would rule there is no contract. There are circumstances under which a court is likely to rule that a contract is enforceable regardless of the fact that mistakes were made by the offeror, offeree, or both. An *attorney* should be able to advise you about whether you are likely to be successful in escaping from a contractual relationship that you entered because of a mistake.

While a court may release you from fulfilling a contract that did not involve a true "meeting of minds," it is unlikely to release you from one you accepted but later found to be *disadvantageous* after studying it carefully. The courts ordinarily will rule that a person has the obligation to study an offer carefully before accepting it (e.g., before signing a contract). While not considering an offer more carefully before accepting it may have been a mistake, a court is unlikely to declare a contract unenforceable for this reason.

Duress The acceptance of an offer is supposed to be a *voluntary* act. A person is supposed to accept an offer because he or she rightly or wrongly views it as advantageous to do so. If a person accepts an offer because he actually or figuratively has "a gun held to his head," the courts are likely to rule that the offer was accepted under duress and, hence, the contract is void *unless the person accepting it wishes it to be enforced.* A person who forces someone to accept an offer may end up outsmarted because the contract may unexpectedly prove to be highly advantageous to the offeree. The offeree can insist on enforcement of the contract in such a case and sue the offeror for breach of contract if he or she fails to do what was promised. Such a situation would be one in which poetic justice prevailed.

The Offer Is Unconscionable Occasionally, a contract contains a clause (or clauses) that is so *unreasonably favorable* to the interests of one of the parties that a judge is likely to rule that the clause is unenforceable as it stands. A judge would be unlikely to rule part of a contract unconscionable unless it *unequivocally* violated his or her sense of fairness (see the discussion of natural law in Chapter 1). Being unconscionable is something beyond one party's bargaining more successfully and as a result getting a better deal. Judges tend to be unwilling to rule parts of contracts unconscionable unless the evidence is overwhelming.

Why would a person accept an offer having unconscionable aspects? The only reason probably would be that he or she had *no choice*. A person who has a desperate need to borrow money but cannot borrow from a bank because of a poor credit rating may be forced to borrow from a loan shark at an extremely high interest rate. In the unlikely event that the loan shark sued the person for breach of contract for failure to pay the exorbitant interest rate agreed to, the judge probably would rule that the interest rate was unconscionable and, hence, the contract was unenforceable in its present form. The judge probably would reduce the interest rate to one which he felt was fair in order to make the contract enforceable.

Illegality The courts will not enforce a contract that violates either criminal or civil law—that is, one that would result in the commission of a crime or a tort. (See Chapter 6 for a discussion of torts.)

The Contract Is Not in Written Form It certainly is desirable for almost any contract to be written, and for some types of contracts it is *necessary*. The courts will not enforce some types of contracts unless they are written. Included here are contracts for the sale of goods over a certain price (which varies from state to state). Also included are contracts that take more than a specified period of time to complete (time periods also vary from state to state).

Possible Remedies for a Contract That Is Breached

What options do you have if a person with whom you have a contract refuses to do as promised? You would have two options. The first would be to seek an *out-of-court settlement* and the second would be to sue for *breach of contract*. Most wronged parties initially would seek an out-of-court settlement; if this were not attainable, they would consider suing for breach of contract. Out-of-court settlements tend to cost less in legal fees than in-court suits.

The wronged party's *objective,* regardless of whether he or she is seeking an out-of-court or an in-court settlement, is *to attain the position he or she would have been in if the contract had been completed.* The most direct way that the wronged party can be put in this position is for the party who has breached the contract to do voluntarily what was promised because the *cost* of not doing so would be too high. The term *cost* here refers not only to time and money, but also to such intangibles as *damage to one's reputation.* Other ways that a wronged party can be put in this position are by having the breaching party return what he or she received as consideration (i.e., by having him or her make *restitution)* or by having the breaching party pay money (i.e., *compensatory damages)* to offset the losses sustained by the contract's not being completed.

Out-of-Court Settlements Before initiating a suit the wronged party to a contract will probably attempt to motivate the breaching party to do as promised, or to return whatever was given as payment for doing what was promised, or to pay an amount of money that would compensate for any losses the wronged party sustained. To achieve this objective he or she may employ such motivational devices as a *letter from an attorney* which makes a direct or indirect threat to sue if the matter cannot be settled out of court. He or she may also threaten to *file a complaint* with an organization such as the *Better Business Bureau* if the matter is not resolved in a satisfactory manner. Such a threat is often adequate to motivate the breaching party to behave in an equitable manner.

Suits for Breach of Contract A suit for breach of contract is a civil suit and is conducted in the same manner as any other civil suit. The procedures by which such suits are initiated and conducted are described in Chapter 2. The plaintiff (the wronged party) may seek any of a number of *remedies* from the court. The one that plaintiffs seek most often in breach of contract suits is *compensatory damages.* This consists of an award of money (from the defendant) that is intended to put the plaintiff in the financial position he or she would have been in if the contract had been completed.

CONTRACTUAL ASPECTS OF THE CLIENT-CLINICIAN RELATIONSHIP

The client-clinician relationship is, among other things, a contractual relationship. The offeror is the clinician and the offeree is the client or his or her family. (Throughout this discussion the term *client* will be assumed to include the client's family where relevant.) The consideration offered by the clinician is time and expertise. That offered by the client is a promise to pay a fee for services received. The client may or may not be aware of the amount of this fee when treatment is begun. In some cases the fee is paid, partially or completely, by a third party such as a public school system or a governmental insurance program. The clinician *offers* a service to the client, which the client *accepts*. The client is likely to conclude that the clinician has lived up to the contract if the client receives from the clinician what he or she *thought* the clinician promised.

The problem most frequently encountered is probably that the client and the clinician have *different interpretations* of the offer. The client when accepting the offer is interpreting it to be what he or she *wants* it to be rather than what the clinician *intends* it to be. Offeror and offeree here do not have a true "meeting of minds." Aside from the legal implications of this situation, it can adversely affect the therapy process.

One way that clients can misconstrue a clinician's offer is to interpret it as *guaranteeing* some level of improvement. They may assume that the clinician by offering his or her services is *implicitly* promising that therapy will result in significant improvement. The clinician, of course, cannot make such a promise for any of several reasons, including the fact that it would violate the professional code of ethics (see Chapter 5). It is crucial, therefore, for both the client and the client's family to understand *when therapy is initiated* that a specific level of improvement cannot be guaranteed. However, some estimate of the likelihood of various levels of improvement should be provided.

Another way by which a client and the client's family can misconstrue a clinician's offer is by assuming that the responsibility for the client's improving rests completely, or almost completely, on the clinician. They may expect the clinician to do things to the client that will cause the client to change in the manner they desire. Considering the nature of the therapy process, such an attitude is not realistic. Speech-language pathologists and audiologists almost always attempt to help their clients help themselves. The client is expected to assume an active rather than a passive role. It is crucial, therefore, that when therapy is offered the client and the family be informed as specifically as possible about what the client would be expected to do and what the clinician would do if therapy were undertaken. Clients should be told that if they are not willing to do what the clinician would expect them to do, they will probably be wasting their time and money by accepting the therapy being offered.

REFERENCES

BLACK, H. C., *Black's Law Dictionary* (Rev. 4th Ed.). St. Paul, Minn.: West Publishing Company (1968).
CORBIN, A. L., *Corbin on Contracts*. St. Paul, Minn.: West Publishing Company (1952).
FISHER, B. D., *Introduction to the Legal System* (2nd Ed.). St. Paul, Minn.: West Publishing Company (1977).
MEYERS, L. J., *The Law and the Deaf*. Washington, D.C.: Vocational Rehabilitation Administration (1968).
Restatement of the Law: Contracts. St. Paul, Minn.: American Law Institute (1973). Copyright 1973 by the American Law Institute. All quotations reprinted with the permission of the American Law Institute.

5

Professional Ethics and Law

Thus far, we have considered two sources of laws that directly or indirectly influence our functioning as speech-language pathologists and audiologists—regulation of practitioners (requirements for licensure, certification, and accreditation) and contract law. A third such source, *codes of ethics,* will be considered in this chapter. Practitioners in health care fields, including speech-language pathology and audiology, are required to be in compliance with one or more such codes. The failure to do so can result in revocation of one's license by the state or of one's clinical certification by the American Speech-Language-Hearing Association.

You may be somewhat surprised to find an in-depth discussion of professional ethics in a book about *legal* aspects of speech-language pathology and audiology. The reason for such a discussion is that there is no sharp boundary between law and ethics—the two are not mutually exclusive. Our views about ethics and morality both influence the *content* of the laws that make up our legal system and the likelihood of these laws being *obeyed*. Also, an ethical code such as that of the American Speech-Language-Hearing Association, contains prohibitions that are intended to prevent practitioners from committing *torts*, such as slander (see Chapter 6).

The overall objective of this chapter is to increase your awareness of *ethical considerations* in clinical practice and clinical research. The chapter begins with a description of the relationship between law and ethics. Next, the role of ethics (including codes of ethics) in shaping the conduct of clinical practice and research is discussed. The Code of Ethics of the American Speech-Language- Hearing Association is then presented from a historical perspective.

RELATIONSHIP BETWEEN ETHICS AND LAW

Ethics (or morality) influences law, which in turn influences how we perceive behavior from an ethical perspective (see Figure 5-1). Hence, ethics is not an entity that is separate from law but is one of the forces that both has and will continue to shape laws at all levels in our legal system.

Individuals in our society (as in all others) are encouraged to behave ethically (morally) in their interactions with others. We ordinarily try to avoid interacting with persons who we *feel* are not behaving in this manner. This is particularly true for persons from whom we purchase goods and services: We usually attempt to avoid dealing with business persons and professionals who are reputed to be unethical.

What do we mean when we state that someone's behavior is unethical or immoral? First, we may mean that some aspects of the person's behavior do not conform to our internal standard for what constitutes moral or ethical behavior. Here we are not *describing* behavior: We are making a *value judgment* about it. We are saying that it does not conform to what we regard as fair, right, or good. Unfortunately, not everyone agrees on what is fair, right, or good. Thus, the same act can be viewed as ethical by one person and as unethical by another. Also, a person's internal standard for what is fair, right, or good may not remain constant over time. A person may view a given act as ethical at one time and as unethical at another. In addition, a person's internal standard for what is fair, right, or good may vary on a *situational* basis. Thus, a person may view a given act as ethical in one situation and as unethical in another.

Second, when we state that someone's behavior is unethical or immoral, we may mean it is *reputed* to be unethical or immoral. Here we are accepting someone else's value judgment. We are implicitly assuming that another's internal standard

FIGURE 5-1 Relationship between ethics and law.

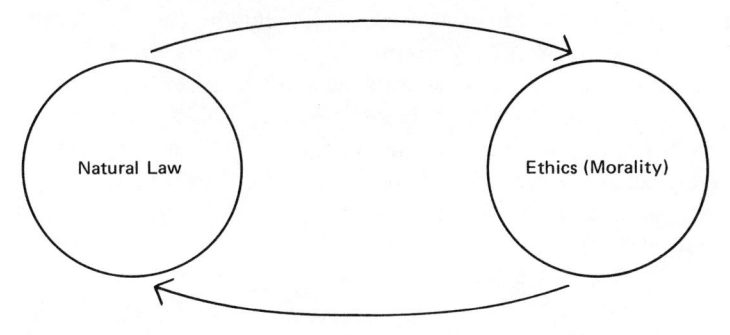

for what is fair, right, or good is the same as ours, which may or may not be true. The situation in some instances is even more uncertain because the judgment being communicated is based not on the experience of the person communicating it but on that of someone else. The person is merely reporting what he or she was told.

The *natural law* tradition is the primary avenue through which ethics influence Western legal thought (see Figure 5-1). Although philosophers are not in full agreement about what constitutes natural law, there are some common elements in the ways that they view it. According to Brody,

> what they have in common is a belief in a body of laws governing all people at all times and in a source for those laws other than the customs and institutions of a given society. Such beliefs are frequently accompanied by the additional beliefs that *no societies are authorized to create laws that conflict directly with natural laws, and that such conflicting laws may therefore be invalid* [italics mine]. In short, the natural law tradition asserts the existence of a set of laws whose status as laws is based on their moral status. (Brody, 1978, pp. 817-818)

Hence, we use our concept of what is ethical, or moral, both as a standard for assessing the fairness of existing laws and as a guide when encouraging legislators through lobbying (see Chapter 12) to enact new laws. If the majority of the voters in a political unit (a municipality, state, or country) regard an existing law as unfair, they may be able to have it removed by a legislative act. Or if a vocal minority of the voters in a political unit regard an existing situation as unfair, they may be able to convince the members of the appropriate legislature of this unfairness, which may motivate them to pass a law that would at least partially rectify the situation. Parent groups have used this mechanism to motivate legislatures to pass laws that provide appropriate special education, including speech-language pathology and audiology services, for handicapped children.

Thus far in this discussion, ethics has been viewed as a *shaper of law.* The relationship between ethics and law can also be viewed in another way. From this second perspective it can be argued that *ethics is law*—in fact, the *highest* level of law. Hence, it follows that laws enacted by government should not be obeyed if obeying them would result in acts that are immoral—that is, contrary to natural law. Such laws, because they violate natural law, are regarded as *invalid*. One can, in fact, be punished by a court for obeying them. This actually occurred at the Nuremberg trials following World War II. A number of persons in postwar Germany were tried for genocide and convicted. It was argued at these trials that the laws that resulted in the Holocaust violated natural law and, hence, should not have been obeyed. Of course, refusing to obey a law because it violates one's sense of fairness may not be accepted as adequate justification by a court. (For further information about the relationship between ethics and law, see the article by Brody, 1978, in the *Encyclopedia of Bioethics*.)

ETHICS AND THE CLINICIAN

Ethical considerations impose restrictions and obligations on the professional activities of a clinician, both those associated with the *delivery of clinical services* and those associated with *clinical research*. These are imposed in two main ways. The first is through the ethical values that all of us began to learn as children and that govern all aspects of our functioning. Some of these are likely to be associated with the Judeo-Christian tradition. And the second is through a *code of professional ethics* (or codes of professional ethics) that the clinician agreed to accept. He or she may have agreed to accept such a code because doing so was a requirement for certification or licensure. If this were the reason, failure to abide by the code could result in loss of certification or licensure.

We will consider in this section the roles played by codes of professional ethics in regulating clinical functioning. The intent is to provide a *philosophical perspective* that should help speech-language pathologists and audiologists to understand better the function of the Code of Ethics of the American Speech-Language-Hearing Association as well as that of other professional ethical codes they are asked to accept.

Ethical considerations have been of concern to clinicians for at least the past two thousand years (Konold, 1978). Until the nineteenth century, almost all clinicians were physicians, and they regarded the prevention and treatment of communicative disorders to be a part of their clinical responsibility. (Some physicians, particularly those living in countries where there are few nonmedical practitioners trained to work with communicative disabled people, still view this as part of their clinical responsibility.) Since the codes of ethics of almost all nonmedical clinical professions (including speech-language pathology and audiology) were based to some extent on codes of medical ethics, much can be learned about ethical aspects of clinical practice by studying the rationales for certain restrictions on the functioning of a physician that are imposed by medical ethical codes and their precursors—oaths and prayers.

Oaths and Prayers

Many of the restrictions and obligations mentioned in medical ethical codes have their origins in ancient prayers and oaths, particularly the latter. The *Daily Prayer of a Physician,* for example, which is one of the better known of the older statements on medical ethics, includes the following:

> Do not allow thirst for profit, ambition for renown and admiration, to interfere with my profession, for these are the enemies of truth and of love for mankind and they can lead astray in the great task of attending to the welfare of Thy creatures. Preserve the strength of my body and of my soul that they ever be ready to cheerfully help and support rich and poor, good and bad,

enemy as well as friend. In the sufferer let me see only the human being. Illumine my mind that it recognize what presents itself and it may comprehend what is absent or hidden.... Let me never be absent-minded. May no strange thoughts divert my attention at the bedside of the sick, or disturb my mind in its silent labors, for great and sacred are the thoughtful deliberations required to preserve the ... health of Thy creatures. (Friedenwald, 1917, 260-261)

The notion that a clinician needs to "hold paramount the welfare of persons served professionally," which is incorporated into all health care profession ethical codes in some form, is acknowledged in this prayer. The ethical content of this excerpt, incidentally, would appear to be as relevant for speech-language pathologists and audiologists as it is for physicians.

Several of the restrictions and obligations that are mentioned in medical ethical codes also are alluded to in medical oaths. The following excerpt from the *Oath of Hippocrates*, which is thought to have been formulated more than two thousand years ago, is representative.

I will apply dietitic measures for the benefit of the sick according to my ability and judgment; I will keep them from harm and injustice.

I will neither give a deadly drug to anybody if asked for it, nor will I make a suggestion to this effect. Similarly I will not give a woman an abortive remedy. In purity and holiness I will guard my life and my art.

I will not use the knife, not even on sufferers from stone, but will withdraw in favor of such men as are engaged in this work.

Whatever houses I may visit, I will come for the benefit of the sick, remaining free of all intentional injustices, of all mischief and in particular of sexual relations with both female and male persons, be they free or slave.

What I may see or hear in the course of the treatment or even outside of the treatment in regard to the life of men, which on no account one must spread abroad, I will keep to myself holding such things shameful to be spoken about. (Edelstein, 1953, p. 3)

The five paragraphs in this excerpt allude to the ethical principle of "holding paramount the welfare of persons served professionally." A pledge is made in the first to use one's clinical skills in a manner likely to benefit one's patients in socially acceptable ways. In the second a pledge is made to not use one's skills to change a patient in socially unacceptable ways, even if asked to do so by the patient. Abortion apparently was socially unacceptable when this oath was formulated. During the twentieth century, it has been socially acceptable at times under certain circumstances. For this reason, contemporary codes of medical ethics do not forbid physicians to perform abortions under all circumstances. This illustrates an important aspect of ethics: What is ethical is not absolute, or unchangeable. An act that may be viewed as ethical at one time may be viewed as unethical at another.

A pledge is made in the third paragraph of the oath to make referrals to other professionals when this is needed to provide the patient with the best service possible. One implication of this pledge is that one should not attempt to provide services for which one has been inadequately trained. Physicians were not trained to be surgeons when the *Hippocratic Oath* was formulated; the practice of surgery was a separate profession. Since all of today's physicians are trained to do some surgery, this ethical prohibition is no longer enforced. This further illustrates the point that ethical precepts are not absolute, or unchangeable.

A pledge is made in the fourth paragraph of the oath to refrain from intentionally doing anything while functioning clinically that will be detrimental to the welfare of the patient. And in the fifth, a pledge is made to not reveal what one has learned about a patient or his family to unauthorized persons. This precept—i.e., confidentiality—is present in some form in all health care profession ethical codes.

Codes of Ethics

While oaths and prayers can have a significant impact on the ethical behavior of those who subscribe to or use them, they are difficult to enforce. The restrictions and obligations that they place on the activities of practitioners are not usually described specifically enough for violations to be established beyond reasonable doubt. Practitioners may be able to claim with some justification that they did not realize what they did constituted a violation of professional ethics. For this reason and several others, the format currently used in medicine and other health care professions for presenting ethical precepts is the code of ethics.

The broad ethical concerns addressed in the codes of ethics of most health care professions tend to be quite similar. The results of a survey conducted under the auspices of Georgetown University's Kennedy Institute and the *Encyclopedia of Bioethics* Project of 525 organizations representing a broad cross section of the health care professions suggests that the typical code exhorts practitioners

> ... to preserve human life, to be good citizens, to prevent the exploitation of patients, to promote the highest-quality health care available, to perform their duties with objectivity and accuracy, to strive for professional excellence through continuing education, to avoid discriminatory practices, to promote the interest and ideals of the profession, to expose unethical and incompetent colleagues, to encourage public health through health-care education, to render service at times of public emergencies, to promote harmonious relations with other health-care professions, and to protect the welfare, dignity, and confidentiality of patients. (Gass, 1978, p. 1725)

The typical code also provides practitioners with ethical guidelines that address such practical issues relevant to clinical functioning as "advertising, billing procedures, self-aggrandizement [i.e., making oneself appear more knowledgeable and competent than one is], conflicts of interest, professional courtesy, public and media relations, employment and supervision of auxiliary personnel, use of secret remedies and exclusive methods, as well as the location and physical appearance of the office practice" (Gass, 1978, pp. 1725-1726).

It should be apparent from this brief overview that the typical health care profession code of ethics contains guidelines and precepts that address most aspects of clinical practice. The remainder of this section is devoted to an examination of several of these that are particularly relevant to clinical functioning in speech-language pathology and audiology. The order in which they are discussed does not necessarily reflect their importance.

Confidentiality One of the most fundamental of all the ethical precepts is the need for confidentiality in the relationship between client and clinician. This need was recognized early in medical ethical thinking as evidenced by its inclusion in the *Oath of Hippocrates*. Originally, this requirement was absolute. Anything that a patient told a physician was supposed to be regarded as confidential and not to be revealed to anyone without the patient's permission. In fact, if a patient told a physician that he was going to murder someone, it would have been regarded as unethical for the physician to inform the authorities. Judging by contemporary medical ethical codes (a representative sample of which are included in the appendix of the *Encyclopedia of Bioethics*), this requirement is no longer viewed as absolute. Information obtained from a patient can be revealed without permission under certain circumstances. The American Medical Association's Principles of Medical Ethics, formulated in 1957 and revised in 1971 (Reich, 1978, pp. 1750-1754) for example, specifies three circumstances under which it would not be viewed as unethical to reveal information obtained from a patient without first securing the patient's permission.

> A physician may not reveal the confidences entrusted to him in the course of medical attendance, or the deficiencies he may observe in the character of patients, *unless he is required to do so by law or unless it becomes necessary in order to protect the welfare of the individual or of the community* [italics mine].

These same three exceptions, incidentally, were mentioned in the 1979 revision of the Code of Ethics of the American Speech-Language-Hearing Association.

The first of these exceptions—being required *by law* to reveal information without the patient's permission—is the one that speech-language pathologists and audiologists are likely to encounter most frequently. Either a civil or criminal court can order them to reveal such information. The likelihood that they could successfully refuse to reveal information requested by a court because they regard it as *privileged communication* would depend on the precedents that govern the decisions of the court issuing the order. If a court previously had allowed similar information obtained under similar circumstances to be regarded as privileged communication, it may be willing to do so again. You should consult an attorney to determine the likelihood that a court will honor your refusal to reveal certain information because you regard it as privileged communication.

The second of these exceptions—to protect the welfare of the individual—is apt to be a difficult one to justify. In fact, a clinician would have to assume the *burden of proof* to justify revealing information about a patient without the patient's permission because he or she thought that doing so would protect the patient's welfare. In fact, revealing such information could result in a clinician's being sued by the patient as well as being charged with violating professional ethics. A speech-language pathologist or audiologist would be faced with this type of ethical dilemma when deciding whether to reveal information from a child client to the child's parents. Aside from possible legal and ethical consequences of revealing information about a client without permission, doing so may have a negative impact on your relationship with the client, who may no longer be willing to trust you.

The third of these exceptions—to protect the welfare of the community—is apt to be extremely difficult to justify. About the only circumstance under which it would be relatively simple for a clinician to do so would be if a client revealed that he or she was planning to commit a crime. A clinician might with some justification feel an obligation to the community to inform the appropriate authorities.

The confidentiality precept applies to both oral and written communication between client and clinician and includes reports and other clinical records. Information in a client's clinic folder should be regarded as confidential, and it ordinarily would be viewed as unethical to release it without his permission. It also would be breaking the law to do so. Legal and ethical aspects of clinical records management are discussed in Chapter 7.

Improvement of Clinical Knowledge and Skills One precept mentioned in all health care profession codes of ethics is "holding paramount the welfare of persons served professionally." This implies that the clinician will use the most effective therapy approaches (i.e., intervention strategies) that the state of the art will allow. The American Medical Association in its Principles of Medical Ethics states that "Physicians should strive continually to improve medical knowledge and skill, and should make available to their patients and colleagues the benefits of their professional attainments." This precept, by implication, places several obligations on a clinician. First is an obligation to keep up to date by reading professional journals, attending workshops and conventions, and taking continuing education courses. The more knowledgeable clinicians are about the state of the art in clinical knowledge and technique, the more effective they are likely to be when attempting to ameliorate their clients' problems. Hence a failure to keep up to date is a serious violation of professional ethics because it is incompatible with holding paramount the welfare of one's clients.

A second obligation of the clinician is to evaluate his or her therapy programs to determine their effectiveness. Doing so would tend to increase effectiveness as a clinician, assuming that intervention strategies that were not having the desired impacts on clients were modified or discarded. To evaluate therapy programs, a clinician must both know how and be willing to do therapy outcome research. For further discussion about the need for clinicians to do therapy outcome research, see Chapter 2 in *Research Design in Speech Pathology and Audiology* (Silverman, 1977).

A third obligation that this ethical precept appears to require a clinician to accept is to advance clinical knowledge and techniques, if he or she has the opportunity. By doing so clinicians improve not only their own effectiveness but also that of other clinicians. One way by which clinicians have met this responsibility is by reporting the results of therapy programs they have used with their patients (while, of course, maintaining the patients' anonymity). Such reports, whether positive or negative, help to increase our understanding of the impacts of intervention strategies.

Truth-Telling and Informed Consent A clinician has an obligation to be honest with patients about the nature of their condition, the prognosis for improvement, and the probable impacts (both positive and negative) of the possible therapy approaches, unless receipt of such information is likely to be detrimental to them. A clinician may also have a similar obligation to the families of patients, particularly when patients are children or severely impaired adults who would be unable to understand the information or on whom such information is likely to have a detrimental effect. The ethical ramifications of telling the truth have been dealt with extensively in the medical literature, particularly with regard to the desirability of informing a patient that he or she is dying. The arguments that have been advanced, both pro and con, have implications beyond this context and, hence, are summarized in this section.

One of the main arguments in favor of truth-telling is that a patient has the right to decide whether he or she wishes to participate in the intervention program recommended by the clinician. Unless a patient has been provided with accurate information about the nature of the condition, its prognosis, and the probable impacts (both positive and negative) of the recommended intervention program (or alternative intervention programs), the patient's consent to participate in the therapy program is not likely to be viewed by a court as legally binding. If a patient is given such information, a court is likely to regard the consent as constituting *informed consent*. The assumption, of course, is being made that the patient can understand the information presented—that is, it is being assumed that the patient does not have a neurological condition such as receptive aphasia, mental retardation, or cerebral arteriosclerosis; or a hearing loss; or difficulty comprehending English because it is a second language. It is also being assumed that the patient is not a young child.

One of the main arguments against truth-telling, especially complete truth-telling, is that it can have a detrimental effect on a patient. If a patient is told that the prognosis for improvement is poor, the therapy may be less beneficial than it would have been if the patient had been given a less truthful or less complete statement of prognosis. Having been given a poor prognosis, a patient may reject therapy or become so despondent that he or she cannot benefit maximally from it.

This situation illustrates a type of ethical dilemma that we frequently confront—one with two possible courses of action, either of which can result in our violating an ethical principle. If a patient is given an honest statement of prognosis, it may have a detrimental effect, thus violating the ethical principle that the welfare of persons served professionally must be paramount. On the other hand, if a patient is not given a truthful statement of prognosis because such a statement would be likely to have a detrimental effect, this would violate the ethical principle that a clinician should be truthful with patients. Confronted by such a situation a clinician has to *weigh* the competing ethical considerations to determine which is the more important.

One aspect of truth-telling that is mentioned in a number of health care profession codes of ethics is not guaranteeing cures. Many variables can influence how much a patient will improve, and a clinician can rarely predict the impacts of all variables with accuracy or how much improvement a patient will make and thus cannot guarantee a cure.

Informed consent is an important ethical consideration not only when providing clinical services but also when doing *clinical research*. Individuals should be fully informed about the potential risks when they are asked to participate in a research project. This topic is discussed in Chapter 10.

Not Exploiting Persons Served Professionally Most, if not all, health care profession codes of ethics implicitly or explicitly prohibit practitioners from exploiting those whom they are serving professionally. Such exploitation can arise from several sources. One is fees charged for services rendered. The American Medical Association's Principles of Medical Ethics, for example, includes the following statement:

> In the practice of medicine a physician should limit the source of his professional income to medical services actually rendered by him, or under his supervision, to his patients. His fee should be commensurate with the services rendered and the patient's ability to pay. He should neither pay nor receive a commission for referral of patients. Drugs, remedies or appliances may be dispensed or supplied by the physician provided it is in the best interests of the patient.

Hence, a practitioner would be exploiting those whom he or she is serving professionally by charging fees that are higher than would be commensurate with the services he or she rendered and their ability to pay. He or she would also be exploiting them by paying or receiving a commission for referring them to other practitioners, by selling them things they do not need, or by charging them for services not rendered.

A second source of such exploitation is accepting patients for treatment or continuing treatment when the prognosis for improvement (or further improvement) is extremely poor. Private practitioners are particularly likely to be tempted to do this if their caseloads are relatively small and discharging or refusing patients will result in a loss of income. By rendering services to such patients practitioners will also be exploiting society if the fees charged for serving them are being partially or completely paid by a third party such as a governmental or private insurance program.

Monitoring Compliance with the Code of Ethics Many health care profession codes of ethics require practitioners to report code violations to the board that monitors compliance with it and to cooperate with this board when its members are investigating the ethical behavior of fellow practitioners. The following statement from the American Medical Association's Principles of Medical Ethics is representative:

> The medical profession should safeguard the public and itself against physicians deficient in moral character or professional competence. Physicians should observe all laws, uphold the dignity and honor of the profession and accept its self-imposed disciplines. They should expose, without hesitation, illegal or unethical conduct of fellow members of the profession.

This obligation is a logical consequence of accepting what is probably the most fundamental of the ethical principles—holding paramount the welfare of persons served professionally. The persons whose welfare you are obliged to hold paramount include not only those with whom you work personally but also those who are served by other members of your profession. For speech-language pathologists and audiologists, this would include all communicatively handicapped persons. Thus, holding paramount the welfare of persons served by members of your profession obliges you to expose the unethical conduct and incompetence of fellow professionals. If you charge a fellow professional with being unethical or incompetent, you obviously must either be prepared to prove it or to provide sufficient evidence to justify an investigation. Otherwise, you may find yourself the defendant in a defamation case.

Patient Selection and Discrimination To what extent is it permissible for clinicians to choose whom they will and will not serve? Is it always unethical to consider race, religion, sex, and ability to pay when making this choice? These questions are answered somewhat differently in the various health care profession codes of ethics. In some, such as the American Medical Association's Principles of Ethics, they are dealt with directly and the clinician is allowed considerable freedom in patient selection:

> A physician may choose whom he will serve. In an emergency, however, he should render service to the best of his ability.... He should not solicit patients.

In others, such as the American Psychological Association's 1972 Ethical Standards for Psychologists (Reich, 1978, pp. 1811-1815), they are dealt with indirectly, if at all. And in still others, such as the 1979 Code of Ethics of the American Speech-Language-Hearing Association (see Appendix E), they are dealt with directly, and clinicians are prohibited from discriminating against clients on certain bases.

> Individuals must not discriminate in the delivery of professional services on any basis that is unjustifiable or irrelevant to the need for the potential

benefit from such services, such as race, sex or religion. (From 1979 Code of Ethics of the American Speech-Language-Hearing Association)

There is one area of possible discrimination that is not currently addressed directly in most health care profession codes of ethics that we should consider here. This is choosing not to provide services (or to provide only limited services) to persons whose bills are paid by third parties such as governmental insurance programs (e.g., Medicare and Medicaid). The fees paid by such insurance programs for services rendered are often considerably lower than those usually charged for these services, and providing services to those covered by such programs tends to entail a relatively large amount of paperwork. Also, the agencies responsible for administering these programs may be relatively slow in paying, which can cause cash-flow problems. This issue is addressed *indirectly* in some health care profession codes of ethics: The American Medical Association in its Principles of Medical Ethics (1957, revised 1972), for example, states that fees charged "should be commensurate with ... the patient's ability to pay." This statement would appear to imply that a patient should not be denied services because the fees that the patient can be charged are lower than the practitioner's usual ones. The ethical issues here are murky, and clinicians will have to rely on their own sense of what is fair, or on the fee policies of their employers when deciding whether to serve such patients.

Advertising Most health care profession codes of ethics place restrictions on the advertising of clinical services. The first Code of Ethics of the American Medical Association (1847), which served as the model for subsequent health care profession codes of ethics in the United States, placed the following restrictions on the advertising of such services:

> It is derogatory to the dignity of the profession, to resort to public advertisement or private cards or handbills, inviting the attention of individuals affected with particular diseases—publicly offering advice and medicine to the poor gratis, or promising radical cures; or to publish cases and operations in the daily prints, or suffer such publications to be made;—to invite laymen to be present at operations—to boast of cures and remedies—to adduce certificates of skill and success, or to perform any other similar acts. These are the ordinary practices of empirics [charlatans and quacks], and are highly reprehensible to a regular physician. (Reich, 1978, pp. 1741-1742)

It would appear from this excerpt that the original impetus for restricting advertising was to differentiate the *trained practitioner* from the *charlatan* or *quack*. (The term *quack*, as used here, refers to a practitioner who lacks the qualifications and training regarded as necessary by proponents of the profession's licensure and certification requirements. There have been at least a few cases in which a practitioner who was viewed as a *quack* was later viewed as an *innovator*.)

Restrictions on the advertising of clinical services have been relaxed somewhat during the past hundred years. There appear to be several reasons why these restrictions were relaxed. First, there is an obvious need to make people aware of who is a qualified practitioner. If only unqualified practitioners are permitted to advertise their services, the public will have difficulty locating qualified ones. Thus, physicians and other health care professionals were permitted to list themselves under appropriate headings in the *Yellow Pages* of the telephone book and to discreetly inform both the public and professionals in the community who may serve as referral sources.

A second reason for relaxing restrictions on advertising somewhat is that such restrictions have been viewed by the courts as constituting *restraint of trade*. From this perspective, restrictions on advertising keep costs to consumers high by eliminating competition among practitioners. If practitioners were to advertise the costs of their services, consumers probably would consider cost when selecting a practitioner. Hence, practitioners would have some motivation to keep their fees reasonable, which, at least theoretically, would tend to lower costs to consumers. Since the advertising of fees for professional services is a relatively recent phenomenon, it is uncertain how much impact it will actually have on the costs of such services.

CODE OF ETHICS OF THE AMERICAN SPEECH-LANGUAGE-HEARING ASSOCIATION

The Code of Ethics of the American Speech-Language-Hearing Association (ASHA) has much in common with those of other health care professions. Like them, it has evolved considerably since its initial formulation (see Appendix E) and will most likely continue to evolve as the law changes and as speech-language pathologists and audiologists are called upon to meet new challenges.

The membership of ASHA has been concerned with ethical issues since the founding of the association in 1925. In fact, one of the reasons mentioned for founding the organization, according to Paden, was "To establish scientific standards and *codes of ethics* [italics mine]" (1970, p.73). The relatively high level of concern that the founders of ASHA had about professional ethics was, at least in part, a reaction to the unprofessional conduct of some practitioners who treated speech disorders, especially stuttering.

> Such persons were known, for example, to make rash guarantees of cure, to require their patients to sign statements that they would never reveal their methods, to charge exorbitant fees, and otherwise to degrade the image of the profession. (Paden, 1970, p. 73)

Also, a few were known to treat speech disorders completely or almost completely by correspondence. Many of the practices that were prohibited in the various revisions of the ASHA code (see Appendix E) were a part of the modus operandi of some nineteenth- and twentieth-century practitioners.

The primary ethical focus during the early years of ASHA seemed to be on preventing unethical practitioners from joining rather than on monitoring the ethical practices of members. This may partially explain why, prior to 1950, association statements about ethics were included in the section of the association's constitution that dealt with membership requirements rather than in a separate document. This focus also is evident from the qualifications for membership that were included in the original (1926) constitution of the association. There were five qualifications listed, one of which was the following:

> Possession of a professional reputation untainted by a past record (or a present record) of unethical practices such as blatant commercialization of professional services, or guaranteeing of "cures" for stated sums of money.

It apparently was not until the early 1940s that the association was called upon to investigate a complaint about the ethical practices of a member (Paden, 1970). (For further information about the development of the ASHA Code of Ethics, see Paden, 1970.)

The primary ethical focus of ASHA at the present time (as it seems to have been since the 1950s) is on monitoring the ethical practices of its members. All members who are engaged in clinical practice and all nonmembers who have ASHA clinical certification are required to agree to be bound by the Code of Ethics. The change in focus from admission to membership to monitoring of membership appears to have come about largely because most persons who joined ASHA after the 1940s had not had sufficient paid clinical experience for their ethical standards to be assessed. Most of those who sought membership during the early years had been functioning as practitioners for a significant period of time, which made it possible to assess their ethical standards prior to admitting them to membership.

The issues addressed in the various revisions of the ASHA code (see Appendix E) parallel those addressed in other health care profession codes of ethics at the same points in time. This has occurred because the health care professions have had to cope with similar ethical problems during given time periods. During the 1970s, for example, a number of these professions had to cope with ethical problems associated with their practitioners' treating patients whose therapy is paid for by a *third party*, such as Medicare or Medicaid. Most of the ethical issues that are addressed in the ASHA Code are discussed elsewhere in this chapter.

Codes of ethics deal with *general principles* of ethical behavior. The application of these general principles to specific situations encountered by clinicians often requires some interpretation. A series of articles has appeared in ASHA publications over the years, some with titles beginning *Issues in Ethics*, that have attempted to interpret how the ASHA Code can be applied to certain situations encountered by clinicians, including the following: *third-party payment* (Bangs, 1970); *dispensing of products* (Ethical practices board interpretations of principles governing the dispensing of products to persons with communicative disorders, 1976); *speech-language pathologists doing myofunctional therapy* (EPB interpretation of "Joint Committee Statement on Tongue Thrust," 1975), *advertising of members' products* (Issues in ethics: Advertising of members' products, 1974); *honoring of contracts* (Issues in ethical practice—Responsibilities concerning the honoring of a verbal or written contract, 1958); *fees for clinical services provided by students* (Issues in ethics: Fees for clinical services provided by students, 1978); *action by ASHA for violation of state association or licensure ethical codes* (Issues in ethics—Ethical practice inquiries: State versus ASHA decision differences, 1978); *speech-language pathologists functioning as audiologists and vice versa* (Issues in ethics: Clinical practice by members in the area in which they are not certified, 1977); *CFY supervisors' responsibilities* (Issues in ethics: CFY supervisors' responsibilities, 1980); *degrees from "diploma mills"* (Issues in ethics: The bogus degree, 1974); *use of supportive personnel* (Issues in ethics: ASHA policy re: supportive personnel, 1979); *public statement by members* (Issues in ethics: Public statement and general announcements: Guidelines and procedures, 1977; Issues in ethics: Public announcements and public statements, 1981); *ASHA members who are uncertified engaging in clinical practice* (Issues in ethics: Identification of members engaged in clinical practice without certification, 1973); *listings in telephone directories* (Issues in ethics: Guidelines for telephone directories, 1974); *gratuities* (Issues in ethics: Gratuities, 1978); and *nonspeech communication* (Nonspeech communication: A position paper, 1980).

The *Ethical Practices Board* (EPB) is responsible for investigating charges of code violations by ASHA members. If the preponderance of evidence following a careful investigation suggests that the member did violate the Code of Ethics, the board can recommend that disciplinary action of some kind be taken. The most extreme action that it can recommend is expulsion from the association. Information about procedures for filing or answering a complaint can be obtained from the ASHA national office. Anyone who has been accused of violating the ASHA code and is being investigated by the EPB would probably be wise to consult with an attorney.

REFERENCES

BANGS, J. L., Third party payment abuses. *Asha*, 12, 418 (1970).
BRODY, B. A., Law and morality. In Warren T. Reich (Ed.), *Encyclopedia of Bioethics*, Volume 2, New York: Free Press (1978).
EDELSTEIN, L., The Hippocratic Oath: Text, translation, and interpretation. *Bulletin of the History of Medicine*, Supplement 1. Baltimore: Johns Hopkins University Press (1943).
EPB interpretation of "Joint Committee Statement on Tongue Thrust." *Asha*, 17, 331 (1975).
Ethical practices board interpretations of principles governing the dispensing of products to persons with communicative disorders. *Asha*, 18, 227-240 (1976).
FRIEDENWALD, H., *Bulletin of the Johns Hopkins Hospital*, 28, 260-261 (1917).
GASS, R. S., Codes of the health-care professions. In Warren T. Reich (Ed.), *Encyclopedia of Bioethics*, Volume 4, New York: Free Press (1978).
Issues in ethics: Advertising of members' products. *Asha*, 16, 44 (1974).
Issues in ethics: ASHA policy re: supportive personnel. *Asha*, 21, 419 (1979).
Issues in ethics: The bogus degree. *ASHA* 16, 212 (1974).
Issues in ethics: CFY supervisors' responsibilities. *Asha*, 22, 273-274 (1980).
Issues in ethics: CFY supervisors' responsibilities. *Asha*, 16, 212 (1974).

Issues in ethics: Clinical practice by members in the area in which they are not certified. *Asha,* 19, 343 (1977).
Issues in ethics: Ethical practice inquiries: State versus ASHA decision differences. *Asha,* 20, 505-506 (1978).
Issues in ethics: Fees for clinical services provided by students. *Asha,* 20, 427 (1978).
Issues in ethics: Gratuities. *Asha,* 20, 311-312 (1978).
Issues in ethics: Guidelines for telephone directories. *Asha,* 16, 708-709 (1974).
Issues in ethics: Identification of members engaged in clinical practice without certification. *Asha,* 15, 381 (1973).
Issues in ethics: Public announcements and public statements. *Asha,* 23, 107 (1981).
Issues in ethics: Public statements and general announcements: Guidelines and procedures. *Asha,* 19, 423 (1977).
Issues in ethical practice—responsibilities concerning the honoring of a verbal or written contract. *Journal of Speech and Hearing Disorders,* 23, 160-161 (1958).
KONOLD, D., Codes of medical ethics: I. History. In Warren T. Reich (Ed.), *Encyclopedia of Bioethics,* Volume 1, New York: Free Press, 162-171 (1978).
Non-speech communication: A position paper. *Asha,* 22, 267-272 (1980).
PADEN, E. P., *A History of the American Speech and Hearing Association 1925 to 1958.* Washington, D.C.: American Speech-Language-Hearing Association (1970).
REICH, W. T. (Ed.), *Encyclopedia of Bioethics,* Volume 4. New York: Free Press (1978).
SILVERMAN, F. H., *Research Design in Speech Pathology and Audiology.* Englewood Cliffs, N.J.: Prentice-Hall (1977).

6

Malpractice and Other Torts

Persons within our society have an obligation, which is recognized by courts, to not act in ways that will adversely affect the physical condition, mental condition, reputation, or property of those with whom they directly or indirectly interact. They have this obligation *regardless* of whether there are laws that specifically prohibit their actions. Ignoring this obligation can result in their being sued for committing a *tort* by a person who was adversely affected by the act. If a clinician, for example, were to use corporal punishment to discipline a child without parental permission, the child's parents could sue the clinician for the tort of *battery*. Or if the use of response-contingent electric shock caused a child a great deal of mental distress, the child's parents could sue the clinician for the tort of *infliction of mental distress*. Or if a clinician told potential patients of a practitioner that he or she was incompetent or unethical, the practitioner could sue the clinician for the tort of *slander*. Or if you entered someone's office without permission, the person could sue you for the tort of *trespass*. Whether the person initiating any of these suits (i.e., the plaintiff) would be likely to win would be determined by several factors discussed elsewhere in this chapter.

The objective of this chapter is to acquaint you with the law of torts, particularly as it relates to the practice of speech-language pathology and audiology. I shall begin by describing some of the basic characteristics of torts. Next, I shall describe some types of torts that can be professionally relevant, including the negligence tort known as *malpractice*. Finally, we shall consider how a speech-language pathologist or audiologist might function so as to minimize the probability of becoming involved in tort-related litigation. Malpractice and other types of insurance that offer one some protection if sued for committing a tort will be discussed.

WHAT IS A TORT?

There appears to be almost universal agreement among writers of books on torts that the term *tort* is a difficult one to define in a completely (or even almost completely) satisfactory manner (Prosser, 1971). One reason is that some of the acts the courts have classified as torts seem to have little in common. Another reason is that the courts through their decisions (see Chapter 2 for a discussion of the lawmaking function of the courts) have classified acts they had not previously classified as torts as being includable in this category. Some of these would not have been predictable from definitions of the term *tort* in existence at the time (Prosser, 1971).

Courts create torts: Acts become torts when they are classified as such by the courts. This may be one of the reasons why it has been difficult to arrive at a satisfactory definition for the term *tort*. Existing definitions appear to have been based, at least in part, on the explanations that judges have included in their decisions for why they have classified the acts as torts. However, the reasons given may not have been their real ones for doing so.

While existing definitions of the term *tort* are not completely satisfactory, they do shed some light on the characteristics of acts that the courts have given permission to be assigned to this category. The following partial definitions that have been suggested for the term *tort* are helpful in understanding this concept:

1. A private or civil wrong or injury. A wrong independent of contract (Black, 1968, p. 1660).
2. A legal wrong committed upon the person or property independent of contract. It may be either (1) a direct invasion of some legal right of the individual; (2) the infraction of some public duty by which special damage accrues to the individual; (3) the violation of some private obligation by which like damage accrues to the individual. In the former case, no special damage is necessary to entitle the party to recover. In the two latter cases, such damage is necessary (Black, 1968, pp. 1660-1661).
3. A tort is a breach of a duty (other than a contractual or quasi-contractual duty) which gives rise to an action for damages (Prosser, 1971, p. 1).
4. A tort is an act or omission which unlawfully violates a person's right created by the law, and for which the appropriate remedy is a common law action for damages by the injured person (Prosser, 1971, p. 2).
5. Broadly speaking, a tort is a civil wrong, other than breach of contract, for which the court will provide a remedy in the form of an action for damages (Prosser, 1971, p. 2).
6. It might be possible to define a tort by enumerating the things that it is not. It is not a crime, it is not breach of contract, it is not necessarily concerned

with property rights or problems of government, but it is the occupant of a large residuary field remaining if these are taken out of the law (Prosser, 1971, p. 2).
7. Included under the head of torts are a miscellaneous group of civil wrongs, ranging from simple, direct interference with the person, such as assault, battery and false imprisonment, or with property, as in the case of trespass or conversion, up through various forms of negligence, to disturbances of intangible interests, such as those in good reputation, or commercial or social advantage. These wrongs have little in common and appear at first glance to be entirely unrelated to one another . . . and it is not easy to discover any general principle upon which they may all be based, unless it is the obvious one that *injuries are to be compensated, and anti-social behavior is to be discouraged* [italics mine] (Prosser, 1971, p. 3).
8. . . . the function and purpose of the law of torts. Contract liability is imposed by the law for the protection of a single, limited interest, that of having the promises of others performed. Quasi-contractual liability is created for the prevention of unjust enrichment of one man at the expense of another, and the restitution of benefits which in good conscience belong to the plaintiff. The criminal law is concerned with the protection of interests common to the public at large, as they are represented by the entity which we call the state; and it accomplishes its ends by exacting a penalty from the wrongdoer. *There remains a body of law which is directed toward the compensation of individuals, rather than the public, for losses which they have suffered in respect of all their legally recognized interests, rather than one interest only, where the law considers that compensation is required* [italics mine]. This is the law of torts (Prosser, 1971, pp. 5-6).
9. The entire history of the development of tort law shows a continuous tendency to recognize as worthy of legal protection interests which previously were not protected at all. . . . It is altogether unlikely that this tendency to give protection to hitherto unprotected interests and to extend a greater protection to those now frequently protected has ceased (*Restatement of the Law: Torts,* 1965-1979, Section 1).

Several general characteristics of torts are indicated by these definitions. First, torts are *civil wrongs* rather than criminal wrongs. They are not crimes. They are wrongs against individuals rather than against society. Hence, in a law suit involving a tort the plaintiff is a person, or a group of persons, rather than a governmental unit (e.g., a state).

A second characteristic of a tort is that it is a civil wrong for which a court will provide a *remedy*. The remedy may be an award of money (i.e., *damages*) to compensate the injured party for the wrong done to him or her, or an order to the defendant to cease doing whatever he or she is doing that is causing the plaintiff to be wronged (i.e., *an injunction*), or something else.

The willingness of courts to provide a remedy for some civil wrongs (such as libel and negligence) is well established. For others, it may be necessary to initiate a suit to establish the courts' willingness to provide a remedy—that is, to establish their willingness to classify the type of wrong done to the plaintiff as a tort.

A third characteristic of a tort is that it is a civil wrong that does *not directly involve the breach of a contract*. The breach of a contract is a civil wrong resulting from the failure of a person to do what he or she *voluntarily* promised to do. (See Chapter 4 for further information about contracts.) The same act performed by a person who had *not* voluntarily agreed to refrain from doing it (by entering into a contract) probably would not be regarded by a court as a civil wrong (assuming that the judge would not regard it as a tort). On the other hand, one is expected to refrain from engaging in acts resulting in torts simply because one resides in a particular municipality, state, or country and by residing there has agreed to obey its laws—tort actions are intended to compensate persons for injuries that they receive because of the wrongful acts of others who reside in the same municipality, state, or country. Hence, the breach of a contract differs from a tort in that the former involves the breaking of a promise that one has made *voluntarily to a specific person* (or a relatively small group of persons) and the latter involves the breaking of a promise that one was *required by law to make to all persons* with whom one interacts (e.g., not to act intentionally in a way that can cause them injury).

A fourth characteristic of a tort is that it results from *interference with the realization of a legally protected desire*. The realization of certain human desires is regarded by the courts to be of such social importance that they are obliged to discourage persons from thwarting them. They do this by imposing *liability* (e.g., damages) on those who thwart or set up roadblocks that interfere with the realization of these desires either *intentionally* or through *negligence*.

What *types of desires* have the courts been willing to protect from being thwarted? There are many (see the multivolume work, *Restatement of the Law: Torts*, 1965-1979), including the following:

1. The desire for *bodily security*—the desire not to be physically harmed or even touched by another without your permission, either intentionally or through negligence (e.g., malpractice).
2. The desire for a *reputation* that is commensurate with your behavior—the desire not to have your reputation damaged by someone's saying or writing something about you that is not true.
3. The desire for your *property* to be secure—the desire for your property not to be damaged, used, or even touched by another without your permission, either intentionally or through negligence.
4. The desire for your *mental state* to be secure—the desire not to have your intellectual or emotional status harmed by another, either intentionally or through negligence.

Some torts that can result from these types of desires being thwarted are described in the next section of this chapter.

TYPES OF TORTS

Most actions that are classifiable as torts can be assigned to one of the following three categories: negligence torts, intentional torts, and strict liability (see Figure

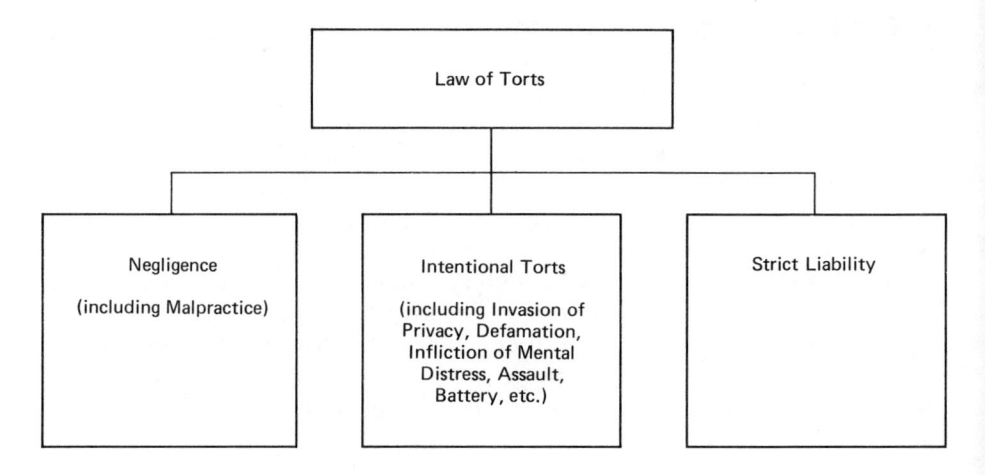

FIGURE 6-1 Classification of torts.

6-1). This section describes some professionally relevant torts that are representative of those in each category.

Negligence Torts

Negligence torts involve carelessness that injures (or harms) others. However, not all accidents are regarded by the courts as torts of negligence. In order for an accident to be so regarded, the following four conditions must be met:

> The actor [i.e., the person causing the accident] is liable for an invasion of an interest of another, if:
>
> (a) the interest invaded is protected against unintentional invasion, and
> (b) the conduct of the actor is negligent with respect to the other, or a class of persons within which he is included, and
> (c) the actor's conduct is a legal cause of the invasion, and
> (d) the other has not conducted himself as to disable himself from bringing an action for such invasion. (*Restatement of the Law: Torts*, 1965-1979, Section 281)

The first and second conditions must be met for the conduct of a person who is responsible for an accident to be regarded as negligent by the courts. The third and fourth conditions must be met before a court would probably be willing to award damages for negligent conduct, once it had been established that it had occurred. If the first two conditions were met but not the third or fourth, the court might agree that the actor's conduct was negligent but would not award damages. Hence, the attorney for the defendant in a malpractice suit may attempt to prove that either the third or fourth condition was not met and, for this reason, damages should not be awarded to the plaintiff.

What interests are protected by the courts against *unintentional* invasion? The

Malpractice and Other Torts

courts have been willing to protect a number of interests against unintentional invasion by reason of carelessness. The following excerpts from the authoritative work *Restatement of the Law: Torts* (1965-1979) indicate some of the types of negligent acts against which the courts have been willing to offer protection:

1. ... acts which are generally regarded as reasonably safe if properly done, the only danger involved in them lying in the chance that the actor may be inattentive, incompetent, or unskillful or that he may fail to make adequate preparation or give adequate warning *(Restatement of the Law: Torts,* Section 297). When an act is negligent only if done without reasonable care, the care which the actor is required to exercise to avoid being negligent in the doing of the act is that which a *reasonable man* [italics mine] in his position, with his information and competence, would recognize as necessary to prevent the act from creating an unreasonable risk of harm to another *(Restatement of the Law: Torts,* Section 298).
    (a) An act may be negligent if it is done without the competence which a *reasonable man* [italics mine] in the position of the actor would recognize as necessary to prevent it from creating an unreasonable risk of harm to another *(Restatement of the Law: Torts,* Section 299). Unless he represents that he has greater or less skill or knowledge, one who undertakes to render services in the practice of a profession or trade is required to exercise the skill and knowledge normally possessed by members of that profession or trade in good standing in similar communities *(Restatement of the Law: Torts,* Section 299A).
    (b) When an act is negligent if done without reasonable preparation, the actor, to avoid being negligent, is required to make the preparation which a *reasonable man* [italics mine] in his position would recognize as necessary to prevent the act from creating an unreasonable risk of harm to another *(Restatement of the Law: Torts,* Section 300).
2. An act may be negligent if the actor intends to prevent, or realizes or should realize that it is likely to prevent, another or a third person from taking action which the actor realizes or should realize is necessary for the aid or protection of the other *(Restatement of the Law: Torts,* Section 305). [Beginning voice therapy before having the client's vocal folds checked by an otolaryngologist may be viewed by a court as such an act.]
3. An act may be negligent, as creating an unreasonable risk of bodily harm to another, if the actor intends to subject, or realizes or should realize that his act involves an unreasonable risk of subjecting, the other to an emotional disturbance of such a character as to be likely to result in illness or other bodily harm *(Restatement of the Law: Torts,* Section 306).
4. It is negligence to use an instrumentality, whether a human being or a thing, which the actor knows or should know to be so incompetent, inappropriate, or defective, that its use involves an unreasonable risk or harm to others *(Restatement of the Law: Torts,* Section 307). [The use of students in training to provide clinical services without adequate supervision may be viewed by the courts as this type of negligent act.]

For further information about the types of negligent acts referred to in these excerpts as well as other types of negligent acts for which courts have been willing to provide a remedy, see Chapters 12 through 19 in *Restatement of the Law: Torts* (1965-1979).

What standard do the courts use to judge whether the conduct of an actor was negligent? This standard, which is referred to in several of these excerpts, is that of the hypothetical *reasonable man*. A person who does not take the precautions when performing an act that a *reasonable man in the same position* would be expected to take in order to avoid harming others is likely to be regarded as negligent by a court if someone is harmed by the act. "Unless the actor is a child, the standard of conduct to which he must conform to avoid being negligent is that of a reasonable man under like circumstances" (*Restatement of the Law: Torts,* Section 283).

If the standard of conduct to which you must conform to avoid being negligent is that of a reasonable man under like circumstances, you should be aware of the *qualities* that the courts ascribe to their hypothetical reasonable man. These are summarized as follows in the *Restatement of the Law: Torts:*

> The words "reasonable man" denote a person exercising those qualities of attention, knowledge, intelligence, and judgment which society requires of its members for the protection of their own interests and the interests of others. It enables those who are to determine whether the actor's conduct is such as to subject him to liability for harm caused thereby, to express their judgment in terms of the conduct of a human being. The fact that this judgment is personified in a "man" calls attention to the necessity of taking into account the fallibility of human beings. (*Restatement of the Laws: Torts,* Section 283)

Deciding whether a person's conduct in a particular situation conforms to what would be expected from a reasonable man in like circumstances may not be easy because it may be unclear how a reasonable man would conduct himself. The attorney for the defendant in a negligence suit is likely to attempt to convince the judge and jury that his or her client's conduct conformed to that of the hypothetical reasonable man and, hence, the *second* of the four conditions that must be satisfied before a court is supposed to award damages for negligence has not been met.

The *third condition* that has to be met before an accident is likely to be regarded by a court as resulting from negligence is that the actor's (defendant's) conduct be the *legal cause* of the harm to the plaintiff. Thus, it is not enough to be able to demonstrate that you were harmed because of the negligence of another. You also have to demonstrate that the negligent act that caused the harm is one for which the courts have been willing to award damages and, hence, has been recognized as a legal cause.

What causes have the court recognized as legal causes? According to *Restatement of the Law: Torts:*

> The actor's negligent conduct is a legal cause of harm to another if
>
> (a)   his conduct is a *substantial factor* [italics mine] in bringing about the harm, and

(b) there is no rule of law relieving the actor from liability because of the manner in which his negligence has resulted in harm. (1965-1979, Section 431)

The defendant's conduct is likely to be viewed as a substantial factor in bringing about the plaintiff's harm if a *reasonable man* would be likely to regard it as such. The attorney for the defendant *may* attempt to demonstrate that while a client's conduct was negligent, it would not be regarded by the hypothetical reasonable man as being the real cause of the harm done to the plaintiff. If the attorney is successful, the plaintiff would be unlikely to be awarded damages.

A defendant can be relieved of liability for a particular negligent act if there is a *rule of law* that relieves persons from negligence liability for that act. A physician, for example, may be relieved from negligence liability for complications arising from an emergency tracheotomy performed on a person who probably would have died otherwise if there is a law that prevents physicians from being sued for harm resulting from such emergency procedures.

The *fourth* and final condition that must be met before a court is likely to award damages for negligence is that *the plaintiff must have conducted himself or herself in a manner that would not disqualify him or her from suing for damages.* A plaintiff can be disqualified by acting in a manner that is *below the standard* of conduct that a reasonable man would expect of someone for their own protection. Plaintiffs who did so would be *contributing to the negligence* that caused them to be harmed. In some states, if the defendant can prove *contributory negligence* on the part of the plaintiff, this will bar the plaintiff from receiving damages; in other states, contributory negligence does not disqualify the plaintiff from being awarded damages but is considered by the court when deciding the amount of damages to award (*Restatement of the Law: Torts,* 1965-1979, Chapter 17).

What constitutes contributory negligence on the part of a plaintiff? According to the *Restatement of the Law: Torts,* contributory negligence can be defined as follows:

> Contributory negligence is conduct on the part of the plaintiff which falls below the standard to which he should conform for his own protection, and which is a legally contributing cause co-operating with the negligence of the defendant in bringing about the plaintiff's harm. . . . Unless the actor is a child or an insane person, the standard of conduct to which he must conform for his own protection is that of a *reasonable man* [italics mine] under like circumstances. (1965-1979, Section 463, 464)

The attorney for the defendant in a negligence suit may attempt to prove that the plaintiff did not protect himself or herself, as well as a *reasonable man* would be expected to under the circumstances and, hence, the plaintiff was negligent.

We have considered thus far the general conditions that must be met before an act causing harm to another is likely to be regarded by the courts as a negligence tort. The remainder of this section deals with the type of negligence tort that probably is of most concern to speech-language pathologists and audiologists—*malpractice*.

What constitutes malpractice? In general, any type of negligent conduct by a professional that causes his or her patient (client) to be harmed either physically or emotionally may be viewed by a court as constituting malpractice. As applied to health care professionals,

> this term means, generally, professional misconduct toward a patient which is considered reprehensible either because immoral in itself or because contrary to law or expressly forbidden by law.
>
> In a more specific sense it means bad, wrong, or injudicious treatment of a patient, professionally and in respect to the particular disease or injury, resulting in injury, unnecessary suffering, or death of the patient, and proceeding from ignorance, carelessness, want of proper professional skills, disregard of established rules or principles, neglect, or a malicious or criminal intent. (Black, 1968, p. 1111)

Society expects professionals, such as speech-language pathologists and audiologists, to exercise reasonable care and to possess a standard minimum of special knowledge and ability (Prosser, 1971). This standard minimum ordinarily is that specified in the requirements for the licensure or certification required for practicing the profession.

The defendants in the majority of professional malpractice suits have been physicians. However, at least a few practitioners in almost every profession, including speech-language pathology and audiology, have been defendants in such suits. Because there is a risk of being ruined financially by a malpractice suit, almost all professionals have malpractice insurance. If speech-language pathologists or audiologists are employed by school systems, hospitals, or other institutions, their malpractice insurance coverage is *ordinarily* provided by their employers. However, speech-language pathologists or audiologists who are engaged in private practice either full- or part-time will have to arrange for their own malpractice insurance. Malpractice insurance currently is available through the American Speech-Language-Hearing Association.

What types of conduct by a speech-language pathologist or audiologist could lead to a malpractice suit? There are a number of scenarios that could lead to such a suit, including the following:

1. A speech-language pathologist accepts for voice therapy a person who has a hoarse voice and does not insist that he be seen by an otolaryngologist for a laryngeal examination. The person discovers six months later that his hoarseness resulted from laryngeal cancer. He claims that he was harmed because the condition was not diagnosed earlier and that this was due to the speech-language pathologist's *negligence* in not insisting on his having a laryngeal examination before therapy was begun.
2. A speech-language pathologist administers swallowing therapy to an adult

who has been diagnosed as having dysphagia. The clinician does not have suction equipment in the room that he (or someone else such as a nurse) can use if the person begins to choke. The client chokes on some food during a therapy session and dies. The family sues the speech-language pathologist claiming that he had been *negligent* by not having suction equipment available when doing the swallowing therapy.

3. An audiologist inserts an impedance probe into a child's ear without first examining the external canal with an otoscope to make certain that there is no object in the canal that could damage the tympanic membrane if pushed against it. The insertion of the probe results in an object's being pushed against the membrane and damaging it. The family sues the audiologist claiming that she had been *negligent* by not examining the canal before inserting the probe.

Intentional Torts

Intentional torts result from acts that are *intended* to injure or harm others and/or are morally wrong. They differ from negligence torts in that the harm done to a person is not due to carelessness. If I told someone that a fellow professional is incompetent, my *intent* probably would have been to damage his reputation and, thereby, discourage people from seeking his services. If he sued me and I was unable to prove that he is incompetent, the court would be likely to award him damages for being slandered.

The word *intent*, as used in this context, denotes the actor's awareness that his act is likely to have certain consequences. According to the *Restatement of the Law: Torts,*

> All consequences which the actor desires to bring about are intended. . . . Intent is not, however, limited to consequences which are desired. If the actor knows that the consequences are certain, or substantially certain, to result from his act, and still goes ahead, he is treated by the law as if he had in fact desired to produce the result. As the probability that the consequences will follow decreases, and becomes less than substantial certainty, the actor's conduct loses the character of intent, and becomes mere recklessness. . . . As the probability decreases further, and amounts only to a risk that the result will follow, it becomes ordinary negligence. (1965-1979, Section 8A)

Thus, people can be held accountable not only for desired consequences of their acts but also for others that they know are likely to occur.

What *types of acts* are the courts likely to classify as intentional torts? Some of those that are professionally relevant are described briefly in the paragraphs that follow. For further information about intentional torts, see Prosser (1971) and *Restatement of the Law: Torts,* Second Edition (1965-1979).

Invasion of Privacy It has been recognized by the courts that people have a right to privacy—a right to be let alone. Interference with this right can result in the tort *invasion of privacy*. Such interference can take many forms, several of which are particularly relevant professionally.

It can be regarded as interference with clients' rights to privacy to *release information* about them from their clinic folder without their written consent, to use *photographs* of them in clinic promotional material without written consent, to write about them in published case studies *in a manner that makes them recognizable* without such consent, or to allow anyone to *view their clinic sessions from behind a one-way mirror* without written consent. Several forms that can be used for securing the client's written consent are included in Appendix A.

Defamation If someone says or writes something *false and malicious* about you that injures your reputation, you *may* be successful if you sue that person for the tort of libel or of slander. If the false and malicious statement were communicated in *written or printed* form, you ordinarily would sue for *libel*; if they were communicated in *oral* form, you ordinarily would sue for *slander*. The law in this area is quite complex, and you would have to consult with an attorney to determine whether the courts would be likely to award you *sufficient damages* to make a suit for defamation (i.e., slander or libel) worthwhile. You could conceivably win a defamation suit and be awarded only *nominal damages*—for example, one dollar.

Not all statements that have been made about you that you view as false and malicious are likely to be viewed by the courts as being libelous or slanderous. Under what circumstances are they apt to be so viewed? According to Prosser,

> defamation is—that which tends to injure "reputation" in the popular sense; to diminish the esteem, respect, goodwill or confidence in which the plaintiff is held, or to excite adverse, derogatory or unpleasant feelings or opinions against him. It necessarily, however, involves the idea of *disgrace* [italics mine]. (1971, p. 729)

While the statement that an audiologist is sympathetic to the use of sign by deaf persons is likely to arouse adverse feelings against him or her in the minds of those who are against their use of sign and while it may possibly even diminish the audiologist in their esteem, a court would be unlikely to consider it defamatory. A *reasonable man* would be unlikely to consider that it reflects upon the audiologist's character and, hence, it could not cause him or her to be disgraced. On the other hand, a statement that an audiologist is *unethical* would be likely to be viewed by a court as defamatory since a reasonable man would be likely to conclude that it reflects on the audiologist's character and, hence, could cause him or her to be disgraced.

A professional's reputation determines to a considerable extent how successful he or she is likely to be financially and otherwise. Therefore, the courts have recognized that they have a special responsibility to protect professionals against false and malicious statements about their capacity and professional conduct. Speech-language pathologists or audiologists not only risk lawsuits by making false and malicious statements about other professionals, but they also violate the Code of Ethics of the American Speech-Language-Hearing Association (see Chapter 5).

Infliction of Mental Distress If someone *purposely* said and/or did something (or is saying and/or doing something) that caused you to become *severely* emotionally disturbed, or mentally distressed, you could attempt to obtain relief from a court. The relief you would seek might be an *injunction* that would order the person to stop saying or doing what is causing you to be mentally distressed or it might be *damages* to compensate you for the detrimental effects that the mental distress has produced.

The word *severely* was italicized in the preceding paragraph to indicate that the courts are unlikely to compensate you for most things people are apt to say or do that make you upset. The courts assume that a *reasonable man* should be able to keep from becoming overly upset by most potentially irritating things that people say or do. Also if the courts were willing to award damages for insults and most other things people do that upset us, there probably would be so many lawsuits that the civil courts would become hopelessly bogged down.

What types of stress-inducing conduct are the courts likely to compensate you for? According to the *Restatement of the Law: Torts:*

> one who by extreme and outrageous conduct intentionally or recklessly causes severe emotional distress to another is subject to liability for such emotional distress, and if bodily harm to the other results from it, for such bodily harm. (1965-1979, Section 46)

Hence, for the conduct that caused your emotional distress to be compensable, it would have to be such that the hypothetical reasonable man would view it as *extreme and outrageous*. The courts are likely to use the following comment from the *Restatement of the Law: Torts* as a guideline when deciding whether conduct has been extreme and outrageous:

> *Extreme and outrageous conduct.* The cases thus far decided have found liability only where the defendant's conduct has been extreme and outrageous. It has not been enough that the defendant has acted with an intent which is tortious or even criminal, or that he has intended to inflict emotional distress, or even that his conduct has been characterized by "malice," or a degree of aggravation which would entitle the plaintiff to punitive damages for another tort. Liability has been found only where the conduct has been so outrageous in character, and so extreme in degree, as to go beyond all possible bounds of decency, and to be regarded as atrocious, and utterly intolerable in a civilized community. Generally, the case is one in which the recitation of the facts to an *average member of the community* [italics mine] would arouse his resentment against the actor, and lead him to exclaim, "Outrageous!" (1965-1979, Section 46)

One technique used with communicatively handicapped children and adults by some speech-language pathologists and audiologists that may be viewed by the average member of the community as extreme and outrageous is the delivery of *response-contingent punishers*, such as electric shock and time out. The average member of your community (whose views would reflect the attitudes of most juries) is apt to regard delivering electric shocks to a handicapped child as outrageous. It is essential, therefore, that *written consent* be obtained from clients or their families before beginning to use a behavior modification approach involving response-contingent punishment. The *rationale* for using the approach and the *risks* involved should be explained to the client's family and possibly to the client so that their written consent is likely to be viewed by a court as *informed consent.*

Assault If others by their actions and/or words caused you to become *apprehensive* about being harmed by them (that is, if they threaten to harm you), you can sue them for the tort of assault. Assault does not involve actual undesired physical contact, only a threat of such contact. This tort is actually a special case of *infliction of mental distress*—the mental distress being caused by a threat of physical harm.

Battery If someone *intentionally touched you without your permission* (even if the contact resulted in no physical injury such as would ordinarily be the case for a kiss), you could sue them for the tort of battery. The courts will protect your right to freedom from *intentional and unpermitted physical contacts* (Prosser, 1971).

This tort differs from assault in that there is actual physical contact. If someone both made you apprehensive about being physically harmed and intentionally physically touched you, you could sue them for both *assault and battery*.

Since plaintiffs in a suit for battery do not have to prove that they were physically harmed—only that they were touched without permission—this tort could have implications for clinicians. Touching a client without permission could lead to being sued for battery. While few clients are likely to even consider initiating such a suit, a clinician should be aware of the possibility and refrain from touching a client who seems like the "suing kind." Obviously, such a suit could seriously damage a clinician's reputation.

Strict Liability

In both negligence torts and intentional torts, a plaintiff is awarded damages because the conduct of the defendant was in some way *faulty*. When suing for these types of torts a plaintiff must establish that the negligence or purposeful conduct of a defendant was responsible for the harm done to him or her before a court will award damages.

In some cases, the fact that the plaintiff was harmed by the defendant will be sufficient to cause the court to award the plaintiff damages. According to Prosser,

> ... the last hundred years have witnessed the overthrow of the doctrine of "never any liability without fault," even in the legal sense of departure from reasonable standards of conduct. It has seen a general acceptance of the principle that in some cases the defendant may be held liable, although he is

not only charged with no moral wrongdoing, but has not even departed in any way from a reasonable standard of intent or care.... This new policy frequently has found expression where the defendant's activity is unusual and abnormal in the community, and the danger which it threatens to others is unduly great—and particularly where the danger will be great even though the enterprise is conducted with every possible precaution. (1971, p. 494)

Thus, an industrial firm could be held responsible for certain hearing losses of its employees because they are exposed to extremely high levels of noise even though the firm took "every possible precaution."

TORT LITIGATION AND THE SPEECH-LANGUAGE PATHOLOGIST AND AUDIOLOGIST

Speech-language pathologists and audiologists, like practitioners in other health-related professions, run a risk of becoming involved in tort-related litigation. Since such litigation can have a disastrous impact on both the practitioners' finances and their reputations, they should do everything they can to minimize the risk. They can do this by increasing their awareness of events that can occur in their interactions with clients and client's families that could lead to such litigation and then taking appropriate precautions. When audiologists and speech-language pathologists are uncertain whether the precautions they are taking are adequate, they would be wise to consult with an attorney.

The risk of being sued for a tort can be minimized, but it cannot be eliminated entirely. It is important, therefore, to have adequate *professional liability insurance*. It may be provided by your employer or you may have to purchase it yourself. An insurance agent who specializes in this kind of insurance can help you determine both the amount and type of coverage that you need. The American Speech-Language-Hearing Association offers professional liability insurance to members desiring it.

REFERENCES

BLACK, H. C., *Black's Law Dictionary* (Rev. 4th Ed.). St. Paul, Minn.: West Publishing Company (1968).

PROSSER, W. L., *Law of Torts* (4th Ed.). St. Paul, Minn.: West Publishing Company (1971).

Restatement of the Law: Torts (2nd Ed.). St. Paul, Minn.: American Law Institute (1965-1979). Copyright 1965 by the American Law Institute. All quotations reprinted with the permission of the American Law Institute.

7

Records Management

All speech-language pathologists and audiologists keep various types of records, including information about persons who have received or are receiving clinical services. Such information may be recorded on sheets of paper, on audiotape or videotape, or on photographic film (such as microfilm), or it may be stored in a computer. Although the needs of the clinician are the primary determiners of what information is collected and how it is used, the law does place restrictions (directly or indirectly) on both the kinds of information that can be collected and how it can be used. In this chapter I shall indicate some aspects of records management on which there are restrictions. Since interpretations of the laws that impose such restrictions are likely to change from time to time because of new court decisions (see the discussion of *stare decisis* in Chapter 2), the specific restrictions that were imposed when this chapter was written are not presented in detail.

What laws govern the management of clinical records of speech-language pathologists and audiologists is determined, at least partially, by the type of setting in which they are working. If they are working in an *educational* setting—such as a college or a public school—the relevant laws will be those for the management of school records. If they are working in a *medical* setting—such as a hospital or nursing home—the relevant laws will be those for the management of medical records. Thus, speech-language pathologists or audiologists can obtain up-to-date information about relevant laws by studying guidelines for records management in the type of setting in which they are employed.

We shall begin by considering the kinds of clinical information, or data, that the courts are likely to regard as records. We then shall consider some aspects of records management on which there are legal restrictions, including record *content* and documentation, record *storage* and confidentiality, *ownership* of records, *access* of clients and their families to records, *correcting errors* in records, record *retention* and statutes of limitation, *transfer of information* at the request of the client or client's family, *requests for information* by someone other than the client or client's family; and the use of client records for *research*. My objective here is to highlight aspects of records management about which you should be concerned rather than to provide specific guidelines. An attorney who is retained by your employer should be able to provide such guidelines.

KINDS OF DATA REGARDED BY THE COURTS AS BEING PART OF A CLINIC RECORD

A record is *an account of what has been done* (Black, 1968). Although such an account usually is written or printed on sheets of paper, it may be recorded on microfilm or stored in a computer. It also may be conveyed, at least partially, by means of recordings (e.g., pretherapy and posttherapy speech samples) or photographs.

Almost any kind of data that helps to tell the story of what was done to a person while he or she was receiving clinical services at a particular institution (e.g., a public school or a hospital) may be regarded by a court as being a part of his or her clinic record and, hence, can be requested (by a *court order* or *subpoena*) as evidence. Included here would be evaluation and progress reports, case histories, clinician's notes about what transpired during particular sessions and telephone conversations, forms on which test results are recorded, and pretherapy and posttherapy tapes.

SOME ASPECTS OF CLINICAL RECORDS MANAGEMENT ON WHICH THERE ARE LEGAL RESTRICTIONS

The clinical record systems maintained by speech-language pathologists and audiologists are required by law to be managed in certain ways. Some of the means through which the law imposes restrictions and obligations on the management of such systems will be indicated in this section.

Record Content and Documentation

The specific types of information that speech-language pathologists and audiologists are expected to collect on the persons to whom they provide clinical services are partially determined by regulations promulgated by state and/or federal administrative agencies, including state departments of education and federal agencies such as the Social Security Administration (which administers the Medicare and Medicaid programs). These agencies influence record content by demanding certain types of *documentation* on those persons for whose clinical services they are at least partially paying.

If a clinician does not collect the information an agency requires for documenting what has been done to a client, he or she will obviously be unable to provide the documentation, which could result, for example, in the employer's not being paid for the services. This would not endear the clinician to his or her employer, regardless of whether the institution was a public school, hospital, rehabilitation center, or nursing home. Clinicians would be wise, therefore, to check periodically with their administrators to make certain that they are collecting all of the information required for documenting their services and for the various other purposes for which documentation is needed.

Record Storage and Confidentiality

One factor that a speech-language pathologist or audiologist must take into consideration when establishing a clinical record storage system is that of providing adequate safeguards for keeping the information stored in it confidential. It has been recognized since ancient times (see the *Oath of Hippocrates,* which is reproduced in Chapter 5) that information a clinician learns about a patient is confidential and *ordinarily* not to be divulged to anyone without the patient's permission. This obligation is recognized in the 1979 Revision of the Code of Ethics of the American Speech-Language-Hearing Association (see Appendix E):

> Individuals must not reveal to unauthorized persons any professional or personal information obtained from the person served professionally, unless required by law or unless necessary to protect the welfare of the person or the community.

Obviously, this prohibition applies to *written* as well as oral communication.

One of the first decisions that has to be made when designing confidentiality safeguards for a clinical record system is to decide *who is authorized to see the records.* Persons who would be so authorized, of course, would include the client's clinician and others whom the client indicated in writing that he wished to see the records. They also would include those associated with the particular institution whom the hypothetical *reasonable man* would regard as having a good reason for seeing them—for example, administrative personnel responsible for billing.

Another group who *may* have good reason to see clients' records are students in training who are observing clinical services being dispensed. This group is of particular concern to administrators of university speech and hearing clinics. It is a common practice at many such clinics to allow undergraduates to see the folders of persons whose therapy they are observing. These folders can contain information that our hypothetical reasonable man would not feel such students have good reason to see. Clinicians would be wise, therefore, to give student observers access only to that data which a reasonable man would feel the students have good reason to see. They also would be wise to obtain their clients' (and/or their clients' families') *written permission* to make this information available to student observers.

To assist both in preserving the confidentiality of clients' records and in documenting who had access to them, the procedures should require persons who wish to see records to sign a dated form and fill in their reasons for wanting access to the records. This procedure would assist in preserving the confidentiality of records by discouraging viewing by persons who do not have a legitimate reason for doing so. It also would provide the data necessary for documenting who had access to records if this information was requested by a court.

For further information about legal aspects of record storage and confidentiality, see Annas (1975, Chapters 10 and 11); Hayt, Hayt, and Groeschel (1972, Chapter 47); and Levine and Cary (1977, Chapter 10).

Ownership of Records

Do a client's records legally belong to the client or to the institution that assembled them for reporting what was done? The answer to this question has implications for several issues, one of which is a person's right to see his or her records.

In most, if not all, employment situations in which speech-language pathologists and audiologists are likely to find themselves, the courts are likely to regard client records as belonging to the institution. The law of all fifty states, for example, recognizes that a patient's hospital record is the property of the hospital (Annas, 1975).

While the institution owns a person's treatment record, it cannot deny the person access to it. As Annas has stated in the context of hospital records:

> Although the hospital is the owner of the record by virtue of custom, and owns the paper on which the record is printed, this still does not mean that it can do whatever it wants with the record. Indeed, there is case authority establishing that while the hospital has a property right in the record, the patient has a property right in the information contained in the record and cannot be denied access to that information. (1975, pp. 114-115)

The question of a patient's right to have access to his or her own records is dealt with further in the next section.

Access of Clients
and Their Families to Records

Clinicians providing speech-language pathology or audiology services in either an educational or medical setting are required by law to show their clients their diagnostic and treatment records if they ask to see them in the appropriate manner.

For those providing these services in an educational setting, the law with which they should be familiar is the Amendment to the Family Educational Rights and Privacy Act (known as the *Buckley Amendment*), which was passed by the Congress in 1974. This amendment guarantees the parents of students the right to examine their children's school records. According to Levine and Cary:

> The major provisions of the law require schools to provide parents of students access to any official records directly relating to their children and an opportunity for a hearing to challenge such records on the grounds that they are inaccurate, misleading or otherwise inappropriate. (1977, p. 110)

This amendment also guarantees students who are over the age of eighteen or attending any postsecondary school the right to examine their own school records. Obviously, any records that public school speech-language pathologists keep on the children they are serving are a part of the children's school records and, hence, subject to the Buckley Amendment.

The procedure that clients or their families would follow to see their records if they received speech, language, and/or hearing services in a medical setting would depend upon the state in which they resided. In those states that do not have laws that enable patients to see their medical records, clients or their families can gain access to them by suing the hospital or nursing home involved and having the records subpoenaed for evidence (Annas, 1975, pp. 116-117). The threat of such a lawsuit is sometimes sufficient to motivate an institution to give a client or family access to the records.

Some states have laws that give patients or their attorneys the right to inspect their hospital records without having to institute a lawsuit *under certain circumstances*. At the time this chapter was written, one of the most liberal of these laws was that of Massachusetts, which provided that a patient's medical records "may be inspected by the patient to whom they relate ... and a copy shall be furnished upon his request and a payment of a reasonable fee" (Annas, 1975, p. 117).

The fact that the law gives clients access to their clinical records has implications for deciding what should be included in a client's folder. You probably should not include anything in a client's folder that you would not want the client or family to see. An example of something you would not want to include would be *negative evaluational statements* about the client's family and their relationship to the client (e.g., "The client's mother seems emotionally constricted and does not relate well to him"). If the client or family saw such comments, their rapport with the clinician could be adversely affected. They may even institute legal action to have the comments removed from the record.

Correcting Errors in Records

A clinician may feel that some aspect of a client's record is in error and may wish to correct it. Because erasures may create curiosity, if not suspicion about the reasons for the change, it would be wise to line out the incorrect data with a single ink line and add the date of the lining out, the signature (or initials) of the person doing it, and the correct information (Hayt, Hayt, and Groeschel, 1972).

Record Retention
and Statutes of Limitation

For how long must a client's clinical records be retained? Legally, this is determined by the *statutes of limitation* for lawsuits involving contracts and torts, particularly the latter. A person is given only a limited period of time to initiate a suit for breach of contract or for commission of a tort (such as malpractice). If he or she waits for a longer time than the statute of limitations allows, he or she will automatically lose the suit. From this perspective, there does not seem to be any need to retain the records of inactive clients for longer than ten years. There may, of course, be other reasons for retaining them longer than ten years—for example, as a data bank for research.

Transfer of Information
at the Request of the Client
or the Client's Family

Clinicians are often asked by clients and their families to send copies of all or part of their clinic records to other professionals. These professionals may be speech-language pathologists or audiologists or other types of practitioners such as physicians. Such transfers of information ordinarily do not create any legal problems if the client or a close family member signs the appropriate release of information forms (see Appendix A).

Requests for Information
by Someone Other Than the Client
or the Client's Family

Speech-language pathologists and audiologists occasionally are asked by somebody other than clients or family members to provide information about clients' communicative disorders, or the services received and their response to them, or their prognosis for further improvement. Persons who might request such information include newspaper and television reporters, employers, insurance companies, government agencies, and attorneys. Before responding to such a request you should consult with an attorney about whether to honor it and, if so, what information to provide. For information about some of the relevant legal issues, see Chapter 47 in Hayt, Hayt, and Groeschel (1972).

Use of Client Records for Research

Speech-language pathologists and audiologists sometimes wish to use information from client's records for research purposes—to answer questions regarding the symptomatology, etiology, phenomenology, prevalence, diagnosis, or treatment of communicative disorders. For some research purposes, such as an individual case study, an entire record may be needed. For others, such as the frequency of occurrence of a particular symptom among persons diagnosed as having a particular communicative disorder, only a relatively small portion of a client's record is likely to be examined and used.

The use of client records for research purposes can be rationalized by arguing that they are being used for "the common good"—that is, for the benefit of society. A client's consent ordinarily is not necessary to use records for "the common good" (Hayt, Hayt, and Groeschel, 1972, p. 1087), particularly if the client's identity is protected. When a client's record is used for research, *"it is not regarded as that of any individual* [italics mine] but as a report involving the study of a disease or group of diseases" (Hayt, Hayt, and Groeschel, 1972, p. 1087).

Although clinicians ordinarily do not have to obtain the permission of their clients to use their records for research purposes, they would be wise to obtain the written permission of the administrator who is responsible for utilization of the record system. The records are the property of the institution and legally cannot be used without institutional permission. For further information about legal aspects of clinical research, see Chapter 10.

REFERENCES

ANNAS, G. J., *The Rights of Hospital Patients: The Basic ACLU Guide to a Hospital Patient's Rights.* New York: Avon Books (1975).

BLACK, H. C., *Black's Law Dictionary.* St. Paul, Minn.: West Publishing Company (1968).

HAYT, E., HAYT, L. R., and GROESCHEL, A. H., *Law of Hospital, Physician, and Patient* (3rd Ed.). Berwyn, Ill.: Physicians' Record Company (1972).

LEVINE, A. H., and CARY, E., *The Rights of Students: The Basic ACLU Guide to a Student's Rights.* New York: Avon Books (1977).

8

Implications of Copyright and Patent Law for the Practitioner and Teacher

Speech-language pathologists and audiologists use various types of printed and audio-visual materials in their interactions with their clients. These include diagnostic tests, intervention programs, games, communication boards, and photographs and drawings intended for eliciting speech. Clinicians also use various kinds of devices—both electronic and nonelectronic—when interacting with their clients. Their *use* of these materials and devices is regulated by copyright and patent laws. These laws also protect the interests of practitioners who develop materials and invent devices for clinical use.

The objective of this chapter is to acquaint you with those aspects of *property law* dealing with copyrights and patents that are relevant to either (1) the *utilization* of clinical, research, and teaching equipment and materials developed by others or (2) the *protection* of your interests in clinical, research, and teaching equipment and materials you have developed. I shall begin by indicating the objectives of copyright and patent laws. Next, I shall describe some aspects of the "new" (1976) copyright law that are relevant to speech-language pathologists and audiologists in their roles as clinicians, researchers, and teachers. Finally, I shall describe some aspects of patent law that are relevant to their functioning in these roles.

OBJECTIVES OF COPYRIGHT AND PATENT LAW

Our federal government has recognized since its beginnings that authors and inventors should be allowed to profit financially from their creations. This recognition appears to have had its origin in natural law (see Chapter 2), which would view it as only *fair* that inventors and authors be granted the *exclusive* right to profit from their creations for a *limited* period of time. The framers of the Constitution, in fact, felt so strongly about the need to protect the right of authors and inventors to profit from their creations that they gave Congress the following power in Article 1, Section 8:

> Congress shall have power . . . to promote the progress of science and useful arts, by securing for limited times to authors and inventors the exclusive right to their respective writings and discoveries.

The mechanism created by Congress for protecting the rights of *authors* was the *copyright*. The corresponding mechanism created for protecting the rights of *inventors* was the *patent*.

Copyrights

What is a copyright? It is the *right to copy* an author's work. The person owning the copyright for a work, who may or may not be its author, has the *exclusive right* for a limited period of time to *make and sell* copies of the work, hence, he holds the *copy right* for the work. The work may be perceivable by vision, audition, touch, or some combination of the three. Works of authorship that are perceivable by vision include books, computer programs, and photographs. An example of a work of authorship that is perceivable by audition is an audiotape recording. And an example of a work of authorship that is perceivable by touch is a book printed in Braille. Examples of works of authorship that are perceivable through more than one sense modality are videotape recordings and sound motion pictures.

Copyright laws have two basic objectives, both of which can be inferred from Article 1, Section 8 of the Constitution (quoted earlier in this chapter). The first "is to foster the creation and dissemination of intellectual works for the public welfare" (Dible, 1978, p. 115). These laws "foster the creation and dissemination of intellectual works" by giving the person who publishes them (who may or may not be their author) the opportunity to recoup expenses and possibly make a profit. They do this by making it unlawful for someone else to make copies of the work and sell them for the duration of its copyright. If there were no copyright laws, publishers would be hesitant to invest the money necessary to publish a work because somebody else could make copies of the work and possibly sell them at a lower price. They might be able to sell them at a lower price because they would not have many of the production expenses of the original publisher such as copyediting and typesetting. (The assumption here is that they would copy the book photographically.)

The *second* objective of copyright laws "is to give creators the *reward* [italics mine] due them for their contribution to society" (Dible, 1978, p. 115). They do this in two ways: first, by requiring anyone who copies part of an author's work to indicate the title of the work and the name of its author, and, second, by protecting the author's right to profit financially (e.g., by receiving royalties) from the sale of copies of his or her works. Nobody is permitted to make and sell copies of an author's works *without his or her permission* for the duration of their copyrights. Presumably, if the author gives somebody, such as a book publisher, permission to make and sell copies of a work, the author will be paid for the privilege (e.g., paid a royalty on each copy sold).

Patents

What is a patent? A patent is "a grant made by the government to an inventor, conveying and securing to him the exclusive right to make, use, and sell his invention for a term of years" (Black, 1968, pp. 1281-1282). This term ordinarily is, *seventeen years.* A patent is not intended to give an inventor the right to make, use, and sell his invention, but (in the language of the 1952 Patent Law) "the right to exclude others from making, using, or selling" the invention. Hence, patents serve the function for inventors that copyrights do for authors. Both "foster the creation and dissemination" of something that contributes to the public welfare (i.e., an invention or a work of authorship). And both "give creators the reward due them for their contributions to society."

PROVISIONS OF THE COPYRIGHT ACT OF 1976

The regulations pertaining to copyrights in the United States are contained in the Copyright Act of 1976 (Public Law 94-553). This was the first general revision of U.S. copyright law since 1909. The act became fully effective on January 1, 1978.

The Copyright Act of 1976 is a complex statute. Because of space limitations, I cannot discuss all aspects (or even all major aspects) of it here. The presentation will be limited to aspects that I feel are particularly relevant to speech-language pathologists and audiologists in their roles as clinicians, researchers, and teachers. The order in which topics are discussed roughly corresponds to the order in which they are mentioned in the statute. (The primary source for this discussion was Dible, 1978, pp. 111-254.)

Duration of Copyright Protection

For works of authorship *created* after January 1, 1978, the duration of copyright protection is the *life of the author plus fifty years after his or her death.* For works by more than one author, the fifty-year period is measured from the date of the death of the last surviving author. All copyrights run through December 31 of the calendar year in which they expire.

Material That Can Be Copyrighted

The 1976 Copyright Act substitutes the phrase "original works of authorship" for "writings of an author" when designating the material that can be copyrighted. Original works of authorship that can be copyrighted under this act are not limited to those that contain written words (i.e., literary works). These also include (1) "pictorial, graphic, and sculptural works," (2) "motion pictures and other audiovisual works," and (3) "sound recordings."

The category of *literary works* includes any works expressed in "words, numbers, or other verbal or numerical symbols or indicia." While a literary work has to be original in the sense of not being merely a copy of a preexisting work, there is no requirement that it be novel, or ingenuous, or possess esthetic merit. Almost any diagnostic or progress report could be classified for purposes of copyright as a "literary work."

The category of *pictorial, graphic, and sculptural works* would include *photographs and drawings* intended for use in diagnosis and/or therapy. Photographs and drawings, like literary works, must be original in the sense of not being merely copies of preexisting images, but their novelty, ingenuity, or esthetic merit are not considerations in determining whether they can be copyrighted.

The category of *motion pictures and other audiovisual works* includes *videotapes* (e.g., videotapes of therapy sessions); the category of *sound recordings* include both *phonograph records and audiotapes.* Again, novelty, ingenuity, or esthetic merit are not considerations in determining whether a work can be copyrighted.

Thus far in this section I have dealt with material that can be copyrighted. What *cannot* be copyrighted? There are six types of material mentioned in the act that are denied U.S. copyright protection. Three of these appear particularly relevant to the interests of speech-language pathologists and audiologists. The *first* of these is *ideas, methods, systems, and principles.* One of the fundamental principles promulgated by this act is that "copyright does not protect ideas, methods, systems, principles, etc. but rather protects the *particular manner* [italics mine] in which they are expressed or described" (Dible, 1978, p. 127). Hence, a copyright does not protect an author's ideas, methods, systems, or principles from being copied; it only protects the particular arrangement of words in which he or she expresses or describes them.

A *second* type of subject matter that is denied U.S. copyright protection is *blank forms.* According to Dible (1978, p. 127), "Blank forms and similar works, designed to record rather than convey information, are not subject to copyright protection." Some of the forms used for recording client's responses to diagnostic tests probably are not protected by copyright for this reason, even though a copyright notice is printed on them. Because a work of authorship has a copyright notice on its does not necessarily mean it is protected by a copyright that has been registered with the U.S. government. Anyone can place a copyright notice on any work he or she creates, including material that cannot be copyrighted (e.g., some test forms). The copyright notice on such a work does serve to discourage others from copying it, simply because most people are not sufficiently familiar with copyright law to know what can be copyrighted.

A *third* type of subject matter that is denied U.S. copyright protection is *works of the U.S. Government.* According to Dible (1978, p. 128), "works produced for the U.S. Government by its officers and employees *as part of their official duties* [italics mine] are not subject to U.S. copyright protection." This category does not necessarily include works prepared under a U.S. government contract or grant. The funding agency can decide whether an independent contractor or grantee will be allowed to copyright works that were supported wholly or partially by government funds.

Ownership and Transfer of Rights

The *author* of a work that was not prepared within the scope of his or her employment is the owner of the copyright on it unless he or she has transferred ownership of the copyright to somebody else. If such a work has *more than one author,* its authors jointly own the copyright unless they have transferred ownership of the copyright to somebody else.

The copyright to a "work prepared by an employee *within the scope of his or her employment* [italics mine]" belong to the *employer* unless the employer transfers it to the employee *in writing.* Such a work is referred to in the Copyright Act as a *work made for hire.* "The rationale for this rule is that the work is produced under the employer's direction and expense; also the employer bears the risks and should be entitled to reap the benefits" (Dible, 1978, p. 130). Your employer, however, would not be entitled to the copyright on a work you authored that was not prepared within the scope of your employment. If you are developing a clinical "tool" (e.g., a diagnostic test or a therapy program) from which you hope to profit financially and if you are doing it wholly or partially at your employer's expense, your employer may feel that he or she is entitled to ownership of the copyright on it. Hence, to avoid a misunderstanding at some later date, you probably would be wise to request a letter from your employer acknowledging your right to copyright the work in your name.

Why might an author wish to transfer his or her rights to a work to somebody else? The reason in most cases would be that an author expected to profit from doing so. A publisher, for example, may agree to pay an author a royalty on each copy of his work sold in exchange for this transfer of rights. An author can sometimes negotiate a contract that allows him or her to retain the copyright on a work and then only sell (usually through an agent) certain rights to publishers (e.g., book club rights). By negotiating this type of contract the author is transferring ownership of a part of the copyright.

Reproduction of Copyrighted Materials and Fair Use

The Copyright Act places certain restrictions on prohibiting the reproduction of copyrighted materials. One such restriction that should be of particular interest to speech-language pathologists and audiologists in their roles as clinicians, researchers, and teachers deals with what has been referred to as *fair use*. For an in-depth discussion of this doctrine, see the Copyright Act of 1976 and Dible (1978).

The doctrine of fair use, which was developed by the courts, "allows copying without permission from, or payment to, the copyright owner where the use is *reasonable and not harmful* [italics mine] to the rights of the copyright owner" (Dible, 1978, p. 142). Without this doctrine, no use of copyrighted material would be possible without the copyright owner's permission. A teacher could not quote from a book or journal article in a lecture without requesting and receiving permission. Or a clinician could not use a diagnostic test reproduced in a journal article with a client without requesting and receiving permission. Or a researcher could not make a copy of a journal article that he needed to consult, without requesting and receiving the author's permission. The idea here is that certain uses of copyrighted materials are not harmful to the rights of the copyright owner and promote the *public welfare*.

What can be copied under this doctrine? Although Section 107 of the act (reproduced here), which deals with fair use, seems somewhat vague, it does provide general guidelines that can be applied to individual situations.

> ... the fair use of a copyrighted work, including such use by reproduction in copies or phonograph records or by other means ... for purposes such as criticism, comment, news reporting, *teaching (including multiple copies for classroom use)* [italics mine], scholarship, or research, is not an infringement of copyright. In determining whether the use made of a work in any particular case is a fair use the factors to be considered shall include—
>
> (1) the purpose and character of the use, including whether such use is of a commercial nature or is for nonprofit educational purposes;
> (2) the nature of the copyrighted work;
> (3) the amount and substantiality of the portion used in relation to the copyrighted work as a whole; and
> (4) the effect of the use upon the potential market for or value of the copyrighted work.

In addition to these general guidelines for applying the fair use doctrine, specific ones have been developed for several areas. One such area is *teaching*. These guidelines permit teachers to make *single copies* of copyrighted materials for use in their teaching. They also permit teachers to make *multiple copies* for classroom use if the number of copies does not exceed the number of pupils in the class and the following restrictions are adhered to:

(1) the copies may not be used as a substitute for anthologies, compilations or collective works,
(2) copies cannot be made of consumable materials such as work books;
(3) the copies cannot be a substitute for purchases, be "directed by higher authority" or be repeated by the same teacher from term to term; and
(4) there can be no charge to the student beyond the actual copying cost. (Dible, 1978, p. 143)

Notice of Copyright

It is *desirable* that a copyright notice be placed on all works for which copyright protection is desired. On *visually* perceptible copies, this notice should contain the following three elements:

(1) the symbol © (the letter C in a circle), or the word "Copyright," or the abbreviation "Copr.";
(2) the year of the first publication of the work; and
(3) the name of the owner of the copyright in the work, or an abbreviation by which the name can be recognized, or a generally known designation of the owner. (Dible, 1978, pp. 228-229)

However, "subject to certain safeguards for *innocent infringers* [italics mine], protection would not be lost by the complete omission of the notice from large numbers of copies or from a whole edition, if registration of the work is made before or within *five years after publication* [italics mine]" (Dible, 1978, p. 165). Hence, immediate, formal application for a copyright is not a prerequisite for placing a copyright notice on a work or for securing copyright protection for it. The mere placement of a copyright notice on a work ordinarily is sufficient to discourage persons from copying it without permission. The formal registration of a copyright, however, does increase the number of types of remedies that its owner can seek from a court.

Deposit and Registration of the Work for Which Copyright Protection Is Sought

The formal copyrighting of a work ordinarily involves (1) depositing *two* complete copies in the Library of Congress and (2) completing an application for copyright registration and paying the required fee. While depositing the two copies of the work in the Library of Congress is not a prerequisite for securing copyright protection, failure to do so can result in your being fined unless *fewer than five* copies of the work have been published or the work is an *expensive limited edition* with numbered copies for which the requirement to deposit two copies would be burdensome, unfair, or unreasonable (see Section 407C of the 1976 Copyright Act). A slide-tape presentation or a videotape production that a speech-language pathologist or audiologist publishes in a limited edition *may* be exempt from the deposit requirement.

Copyright Infringement and Remedies

Owners of a copyright can seek several types of remedies from a court if the copyright is infringed. They can ask the court to issue an *injunction* or *restraining order* that will temporarily or permanently prevent or stop infringements. They can ask the court to *impound* all allegedly infringing copies of the work during the time a suit for infringement is pending. They can ask the court to award *actual damages,* which would compensate them for the profits they lost because of the sale of the infringer's copies. Or they can ask the court to award them *statutory damages,* which are a type of punitive damages (see Chapter 2) that defendants can be required to pay simply because they infringed the plaintiff's copyright. They are referred to as *statutory* damages because they are specified in the statute, or law.

PROVISIONS OF U.S. PATENT LAW

The regulations pertaining to U.S. patents, when this chapter was written, were contained in the 1952 Revision of the Patent Law, which came into effect on January 1, 1953. This law is quite complex, and it will not be possible to give an in-depth presentation on it here. The law is reprinted in a pamphlet entitled *Patent Laws,* which is sold by the U.S. Goverment Printing Office, and it is discussed in Dible (1978).

Subject Matter That Can Be Patented

Practically anything *new and useful* that is made as well as practically any *new process* for making useful things is patentable. The law states that any person who "invents or discovers any new and useful process, machine, manufacture, or composition of matter, or any new and useful improvements thereof, may obtain a patent." Hence, a speech-language pathologist or audiologist who invents a *new and useful* device for evaluating or treating the communicatively handicapped could apply for and probably obtain a patent for it. Such devices would include new or improved types of audiometric testing equipment (or components thereof) and electronic communication devices for severely communicatively handicapped children and adults. A perusal of advertisements in the journal *Asha* and in the programs distributed at ASHA national conventions will provide many examples of *new and useful* devices intended to benefit the communicatively handicapped.

The term *useful* as applied to devices on which patents are sought has a specific meaning. According to Dible:

> The term "useful" in this connection refers to the condition that the subject matter has a useful purpose and also includes operativeness, that is, a machine which will not operate to perform the intended purpose would not be called useful. (1978, p. 3)

Hence, when you apply for a patent on a device, you must be able to demonstrate that it will perform the function(s) you claim it will perform.

The term *new* as applied to devices on which patents are sought also has a specific meaning. The statute states that an invention will *not* be regarded as new (and, hence, cannot be patented) if one of the following applies:

> (a) The invention was known or used by others in this country, or patented or described in a printed publication in this or a foreign country, before the invention thereof by the applicant for patent, or
>
> (b) The invention was patented or described in a printed publication in this or a foreign country or in public use or on sale in this country more than one year prior to the date of the application for patent in the United States.

In addition, the invention must be sufficiently different from the most nearly similar thing which has been patented that a *reasonable person* would regard the differences as more than trivial—that is, would regard it as an "invention over the prior art" (Dible, 1978, p. 4).

Suppose that you invent a test or a therapy tool that consists of printed matter. Can it be patented? The courts have held that printed matter cannot be patented (Dible, 1978), although it can, of course, be copyrighted. The same probably would be true for tests and therapy tools that consist of visual images (i.e., photographs and drawings).

Applying for a Patent

The inventor of a device is the only one who can apply for a patent on it, assuming that he or she is alive and legally sane. It is a *crime* for anyone to falsely state that he or she is the inventor of a device and apply for a patent on it. For this reason, any controversy about who invented a device should be resolved before an attempt is made to patent it. Colleagues, for example, might claim that their suggestions contributed significantly to your invention and, therefore, they should share in the financial benefits that you receive from it.

Perhaps the first consideration in deciding whether to apply for a patent is to make certain that the device is practical and sufficiently innovative so that you are likely to *profit financially* from a patent on it. Applying for a patent can be costly in both time and money. Hence, it *may* not be worthwhile to patent an invention that would be unlikely to yield a reasonable financial return.

If you decide to patent your invention, it may be important for you to be able to document the date on which you first conceived of the idea. This can be done by having persons whom you told about the invention state in writing the date on which they first recall your describing it to them and/or the date on which they first read a written description of it. Such documentation can be useful if someone claims to have invented the same thing at an earlier date.

Since an invention must be *new* to be patentable, a necessary step in filing a patent application is demonstrating that no similar device has been patented in the United States or elsewhere. This involves making a *systematic search* of existing patents. This search ordinarily is made in the Search Room of the Patent and Trademark Office. The inventor may make the search or hire a patent practitioner to make it. If the search does not reveal any similar devices, he or she can prepare and file a patent application.

A patent application has several parts. One is an oath in which the person filing the application declares that he or she is the original, first, and sole inventor of the device for which a patent is sought. (The results of the patent search support this declaration.) Another part is a detailed description of the invention and a drawing of it. Ordinarily, an inventor retains a patent attorney or patent agent (i.e., a patent specialist who is not an attorney) to assist in preparing the application and filing it at the Patent and Trademark Office.

After the application is filed it is examined by a Patent and Trademark Office examiner. The examiner decides whether the invention has been properly described and also performs a patent search to verify the inventor's declaration that the invention is new. When the examiner is convinced that the invention is new and useful and that the application has been prepared properly, he or she will recommend that a patent be granted.

Once inventors have been granted a patent they may sell, or assign, the patent to someone who wishes to manufacture and market the invention. They may retain the patent, and license its use by one or more manufacturers. Or they may decide to manufacture and market the invention themselves.

Notice of Patent

A notice of patent must be attached to all patented articles. The notice should consist of the word "Patent" and the number of the patent. A patentee (i.e., one who owns a patent) ordinarily cannot recover damages from an infringer if the appropriate notice was not attached to the patented article in question.

Some articles have the words "patent applied for" or "patent pending" on them. These words merely indicate that a patent has been applied for. The invention is not legally protected from patent infringement until the patent is granted.

Patent Infringement and Remedies

Infringement of a patent is "the unauthorized making, using, or selling of the patented invention within the territory of the United States during the term of the patent" (Dible, 1978, p. 26). The types of remedies that a court can grant for patent infringement are essentially the same as those that were mentioned elsewhere in this chapter for copyright infringement.

REFERENCES

BLACK, H. C., *Black's Law Dictionary*. St. Paul, Minn.: West Publishing Company (1968).
DIBLE, D. M. (Ed.), *What Everybody Should Know About Patents, Trademarks and Copyrights*. Fairfield, Calif.: Entrepreneur Press (1978).

9

Legal Aspects of Administration and Private Practice

The delivery of speech, language, and hearing services to the communicatively handicapped is a *business* and as such is subject to the laws that regulate businesses. That a clinical facility has no prospect of making a profit—as is the case for most facilities delivering speech, hearing, and/or language services—does not exclude it from being classified in this manner (Black, 1968, p. 249). Hence, speech-language pathologists and audiologists are operating a business, regardless of whether they are engaged in private practice or are functioning within an institution such as a hospital or school system. On this basis they are subject to certain state and federal regulations. Anyone who administers a unit providing services to the communicatively handicapped—even a unit employing only one clinician who is also the administrator—must be aware of these regulations.

Some aspects of business law that have relevance for establishing and administering a clinical facility will be described in this chapter. I shall begin by discussing the three types of legal structures (i.e., single proprietorship, partnership, or corporation) that can be used for organizing a clinical facility. Legal aspects of the employer-employee relationship will be considered next, including some types of statutes that regulate this relationship. Legally and ethically acceptable forms of advertising will then be indicated. Finally, the types of records that must be kept for tax and other purposes will be considered.

ORGANIZATIONAL STRUCTURES FOR CLINICAL FACILITIES

Three basic approaches to business organization are utilized by nongovernmental facilities offering clinical services to the communicatively handicapped: individual ownership (or proprietorship), partnership, and incorporation. This section will indicate the advantages and disadvantages of these organizational structures, particularly as they apply to *private practice* in speech-language pathology and audiology.

Individual Ownership

Individual ownership (or single proprietorship) is regarded as the *least complex* of these organizational forms. It is the type that is most likely to be adopted by a speech-language pathologist or audiologist who is beginning a private practice, particularly a part-time private practice. When this organizational form is used, the business (e.g., a private practice) is *owned by a single person.* More than half the businesses in this country are individually owned. The owner may employ other persons, including other professionals. Hence, an audiologist may own a hearing aid dealership that employs a second, part-time audiologist and a secretary. Two advantages of individual ownership are that the owner is responsible only to himself or herself and reaps the profits if the enterprise is successful. Another possible advantage is that the legal costs of establishing a business using this structure tend to be less than when either of the others is used. The main disadvantage of this organizational form is that the owner is entirely responsible for any debts and losses that the business incurs. This would mean, for example, that if a private practice were not successful, the owner would have to pay all persons owed money (e.g., employees and landlord) from personal funds. If these were not sufficient to cover the debts, creditors could ask a court to order that the owner's home and other possessions be sold. Hence, the failure of an individually owned business can lead to the financial ruin of its owner. A person beginning a business may partially for this reason opt for one of the other organizational forms.

Partnership

Partnership differs from individual ownership in that a business is owned by *two or more persons* rather than a single person. Any number of persons can enter into a partnership. Those entering into a partnership invest their money or their services or both. An audiologist could begin a hearing aid dealership by investing his or her services and by locating one or more persons who were willing to invest the money needed for the purpose. Or two audiologists could begin a hearing aid dealership by investing both their money and their services. A written agreement, or contract (see Chapter 4), usually is drawn up that specifies the rights and duties of all participants in the partnership. The partners share equally in both the profits and the losses of the business unless the agreement specifies otherwise. If there are losses, the partners are obliged to pay them from their own personal property. Hence, one advantage of partnership over individual ownership is that the losses (if there are any) are shared—that is, they are not the responsibility of a single person. A partnership agreement may for a limited or indefinite period of time, depending on the needs of the partners.

Corporation

One disadvantage of both individual ownership and partnership is that any losses incurred by a business have to be paid by its owner or owners (i.e., partners) from their own personal resources. Thus, a speech-language pathologist or audiologist who uses one of these organizational forms to establish a private practice not only risks not making a living if the practice is unsuccessful, but also risks having to use personal property to pay its debts.

One advantage of the corporate structure over the other two is that it ordinarily protects the owner(s) of a business from personal liability if there are losses. "A corporation obtains its financing by selling stock, or shares of ownership, and the liability of a stockholder in almost all situations is limited to the cost of the stock for which he subscribes" (*You and the Law,* 1977, p. 509).

The reason for the owners and officers of a corporation having limited personal liability is that a corporation is classified by the courts as a *person*—i.e., an independent entity. A corporation can buy and sell property in its own name, and it can commit crimes and torts and be tried and punished for them. Businesses established as single proprietorships or partnerships are not regarded by the courts as independent entities but as extensions of their owners. Hence, the property of a single proprietorship or partnership is regarded by the courts as belonging to its owner or owners. Thus, the initiating of a court action against a single proprietorship or partnership involves suing its owner or owners.

A corporation acquires its status as an independent legal entity on the basis of how it is formed. "A corporation is a group of people who obtain a charter from the *state government* [italics mine] that grants them, as a unit, some of the legal rights, powers, and liabilities of an individual human being for conducting any lawful activities" (*You and the Law,* 1977, p. 508). The state endows it with perpetual existence. A corporation continues to exist even after all the persons responsible for obtaining its charter either die or sell their interest in it. It does not cease to exist until it is dissolved by the appropriate legal procedure.

A charter for a corporation is granted by a state government rather than the federal government. Ordinarily, a charter is sought from the state in which the owners of the corporation live and in which the corporation will transact a significant proportion of its business. Sometimes, however, the charter is sought from a state other than the one in which the owners live. The state from which they are most likely to seek a charter in such instances is *Delaware.* This is because the tax and other laws relevant to corporations in Delaware are viewed as being more favorable than are those of other states (Nicholas, 1977). While a corporation can function in a state other than the one in which it was chartered, in such a state it probably will be viewed as a "foreign" corporation and for this reason may be treated differently from a corporation that was chartered in that state.

An organization does not have to be large to incorporate. It is theoretically possible in some states (e.g., Delaware) for a *single* individual to apply for and obtain a charter for a corporation. A private practice in speech-language pathology or audiology probably could be incorporated in such a state.

The main *disadvantages* of the corporate structure are (1) it tends to be more expensive to establish (e.g., with respect to legal fees) than the partnership or single proprietorship and (2) the tax rate on corporate income is usually higher than on individual income. However, because of certain deductions that may be possible from corporate income that are not possible from individual income, the corporate structure will not necessarily result in a higher outlay for taxes than the single proprietorship or partnership. An accountant can advise you about the tax and other financial implications of incorporating.

The procedure for incorporating varies somewhat from state to state. For this reason you should consult with an attorney if you are considering incorporating.

LEGAL ASPECTS OF THE EMPLOYER-EMPLOYEE RELATIONSHIP

Most speech-language pathologists and audiologists function as employers, employees, or both. If you are receiving a salary for your services, you would ordinarily be regarded as an employee. If you hire persons and they are paid a salary for their services by you or your institution, you would ordinarily be regarded as an employer. And if you are both receiving a salary and involved in the hiring of other persons, you ordinarily would be regarded as functioning in both roles. Hence, a person functioning as the administrator (part- or full-time) of speech and/or hearing services in an institution such as a public school or hospital probably would be functioning as an employer as well as an employee and, hence, would have to be aware of legal aspects of the employer role.

Master-Servant, Principal-Agent, and Employer-Independent-Contractor Relationships

The specific legal responsibilities of an employer to an employee and of an employee to an employer depend on whether their relationship would be most likely to be viewed by the courts as that of a *master to a servant*, or a *principal to an agent*, or an *employer to an independent contractor*. The legal responsibilities of an employer to an employee in a specific situation are determined by whether in that situation the employer is functioning as a "master," a "principal," or an "employer." The relationship with a particular employee in some situations may be that of a master to a servant; in others it may be that of a principal to an agent or of an employer to an independent contractor. The terms *master* and *servant* as used in this context do not have their usual meanings; their meanings here are more metaphorical than literal.

One of the main differences among these three types of relationships is the amount of responsibility that the employer assumes for the activities of the employee. The employer assumes more responsibility for the activities of the employee in the master-servant relationship than in the principal-agent relationship. He or she assumes least responsibility for these activities in the employer-independent-contractor relationship.

What are the characteristics of a *master-servant relationship?* According to Black:

> The relation of master and servant exists where one person, for pay or other valuable consideration, enters into the service of another and devotes to him his personal labor for an agreed period ... It usually contemplates employer's right to *prescribe* [italics mine] end and direct means and methods of doing work. (1968, p. 1127)

Hence, in this type of relationship the employer (or someone whom the employer has authorized to act in his or her behalf) prescribes not only *what* the employee is to do, but *how* he or she is to do it. A master-servant relationship would exist between a speech-language pathologist and a paraprofessional communication aide if the speech-language pathologist prescribes not only the type of therapy the paraprofessional is to administer but also how it is to be administered.

Because the employee in a master-servant relationship theoretically is following orders, the *person giving the orders* (e.g., the person prescribing therapy) is legally responsible for any damage done to person or property by the employee which resulted from the orders being carried out. Physicians have traditionally had relationships of this type with nurses, physical therapists, occupational therapists, and other health professionals who have worked under their prescriptions. Some recent court decisions, however, have held such persons partially responsible for damage done to patients by a prescription's being carried out. Health professionals are particularly likely to be expected to share responsibility for such damage if they are aware that a prescribed treatment they are administering to a patient is likely to be harmful. Because speech-language pathologists and audiologists ordinarily do not work under a physician's prescription, they are not exempted from legal responsibility for any damage they do to clients.

What are the characteristics of a *principal-agent relationship?* According to Black, an *agent* is

> one who deals not only with things, as does a servant, but with persons, *using his own discretion as to means* [italics mine], and frequently establishing contractual relations between his principal and third persons. (1968, pp. 85-86)

An "agent," therefore, differs from a "servant" in the following two ways. First, an agent ordinarily is not told specifically how to carry out assigned duties but is ordinarily permitted to use "his own discretion as to means." For example, a speech-language pathologist employed by a school system who was functioning as an agent would be told to provide clinical services to children at a particular school in the system, but the particular children he served and how he served them would be left to "his own discretion."

A second way in which an agent differs from a servant is that agents can *establish contractual relations* between their employers (i.e., principal) and third persons. For example, a public school speech-language pathologist who was functioning as an agent would be establishing contractual relations between her employer and a particular test publisher (third person) when ordering a diagnostic test from that publisher for use in her school.

Speech-language pathologists and audiologists who are employed by schools, hospitals, or other institutions ordinarily function as agents. Because clinicians functioning as agents would be exercising some discretion over who they serve and how they serve them, they would have to assume *some* legal responsibility for any damage that they did to their clients. They probably would not have to assume the full responsibility if they committed a tort because a court would be likely to view the employer (principal) as tacitly certifying their professionalism and competence by employing them. Hence, an employer would have to assume some of the responsibility for any damage that a clinician did to a client.

What are the characteristics of an *employer-independent-contractor relationship?* According to Black, an *independent contractor* is

> one who, exercising an independent employment, contracts to do a piece of work according to his own methods and without being subject to the control of his employer except as to the results of the work. (1968, p. 911)

Hence, "independent contractors" differ from "agents" or "servants" in several ways. First, they are self-employed. They contract with their employers to do a particular piece of work. An audiologist, for example, might contract with an industrial firm to screen its employees for noise-induced hearing loss for an agreed-upon fee per employee. The audiologist would not be an employee of the industrial firm. He would be a self-employed professional who was paid a fee to perform "a piece of work" (i.e., a hearing screening). Once the hearing tests were performed, his relationship with the firm would end.

A second way in which independent contractors differ from agents or servants (particularly the latter) is that their employers ordinarily do not specify how the work is to be performed. They specify the desired results in the contract and ordinarily leave the means to the discretion of the independent contractor. To fulfill his contract the audiologist in our previous example would have to report the status of each employee's hearing to the firm. He could use any testing procedure he wished that would be expected to yield audiometric test data possessing adequate validity and reliability for the purpose.

Speech-language pathologists and audiologists in private practice would be independent contractors. As such, they would have to bear the full responsibility for any damage that they did to clients. They would be wise, therefore, to purchase professional liability insurance. Information about where such insurance can be purchased can be obtained from the American Speech-Language-Hearing Association.

Thus far, we have considered the employer-employee relationship primarily from the perspective of the employee. When we consider the role of an employee as a servant, agent, or independent contractor from an *employer's perspective,* one of the main concerns is the employer's responsibility for the employees' work-related torts and broken (breached) contracts. The concept that one person can be held responsible for another person's torts and broken contracts is referred to in the legal literature as the doctrine of *respondeat superior.* "The fundamental rule generally recognized is that the doctrine of *respondeat superior* is applicable to the relation of master and servant or of principal and agent, but not to that of employer and independent contractor" (from court opinion in *Miller* v. *Metropolitan Life Insurance Company,* 134 Ohio St. 289). Hence, employers can protect themselves from responsibility for the work-related torts and broken contracts of their employees by utilizing independent contractors. A nursing home probably could protect itself from tort litigation associated with the delivery of speech, language, and hearing services by contracting with a private practitioner for their delivery.

Governmental Regulation of the Employer-Employee Relationship

Many aspects of the employer-employee relationship are regulated directly or indirectly by both state and federal government, particularly the latter. These include the following: (1) factors to consider when deciding whether to hire, fire, or promote someone; (2) the nature of the physical work environment; (3) the manner in which employer-employee disputes are settled; and (4) the compensation of employees for their services. Some implications of each are indicated in the following paragraphs.

An employer ordinarily is not permitted to hire, fire, or promote employees strictly on the basis of whether or not he or she likes them. A number of laws *prohibit discrimination* in hiring, firing, and promotion on the basis of extraneous (to the requirements of the job) employee characteristics such as age, gender, race, religion, sexual preference, and/or possession of a handicapping condition. Some regulations go one step further: They require *preference* to be given in hiring, firing, and promotion to persons against whom society has discriminated in the past for one or more of these reasons. This is referred to as *affirmative action.*

The government also regulates to some extent the conditions under which work is performed. The main thrust of governmental regulation in this area appears to be the minimizing of hazards to workers' health. One federal administrative agency that has been quite involved with this area is the Occupational Safety and Health Administration (OSHA). An aspect of the work environment that OSHA has attempted to regulate is ambient noise level.

The government has made some attempt to regulate how disputes between employers and employees are resolved. Persons associated with government agencies have been instrumental in arbitrating such disputes. The government is unlikely to become involved in such disputes unless they are viewed as seriously threatening the public interest.

Many government regulations deal with how employees are to be compensated for their services. They deal with such matters as the minimum wage that can be offered to an employee, employers' and employees' contributions to employees' Social Security accounts, and the percentages of wages that must be withheld for state and federal income taxes.

ADVERTISING

Professionals advertise to make potential consumers aware of their services. Speech-language pathologists and audiologists traditionally have adhered to the ethical restrictions on advertising adopted by other health professionals, such as physicians and dentists. Prior to the 1970s, direct advertising of clinical services was restricted to such activities as listing oneself in the appropriate section of the Yellow Pages of the telephone book and placing a "dignified" announcement in local newspapers when beginning a private practice. According to the 1979 revision of the ASHA Ethical Code, such an announcement may include the following: "identification by name, appropriate professional title and qualifications, services offered, fees, location, hours, and telephone number." Indirect advertising consists of such activities as making other professionals and agencies in the community who were potential referral sources aware of the clinical services being offered by contacting them personally or by speaking about these services at meetings they attend.

Ethical restrictions on the advertising of clinical services offered by health professionals were relaxed somewhat during the late 1970s, in part as a result of a 1978 Supreme Court decision *(United States* v. *National Society of Professional Engineers)* in which "the Court found that it was illegal for any professional society to hold its members to an ethical code which had the effect of limiting competition among its members" (Del Polito, 1979, p. 924). An ethical code that placed restraints on advertising could be interpreted as having the effect of limiting competition.

RECORD KEEPING FOR TAX
AND OTHER BUSINESS PURPOSES

A clinical facility is classified as a business, and hence it is required to keep the same types of records as other businesses. The specific types that must be kept are determined, in part, by whether the facility is organized as a single proprietorship, a partnership, or a corporation. It is important when beginning a clinical practice to have an accountant develop a record-keeping system that will yield the information required for meeting municipal, state, and federal statutes and regulations concerned with taxes and other aspects of business management.

ADDENDUM

Further information about the business aspects of clinical practice in speech-language pathology and audiology can be obtained from the American Speech-Language-Hearing Association and from the American Academy of Private Practice in Speech Pathology and Audiology. This aspect of clinical practice is one of the main areas with which the Academy is concerned. *Private Practice in Audiology and Speech Pathology,* edited by Battin and Fox (1978), and *Speech and Language Procedure Manual,* by Lehrhoff and Koroshec (no date), also are helpful in this regard.

REFERENCES

BATTIN, R. R., and FOX, D. R. (Eds.), *Private Practice in Audiology and Speech Pathology.* New York: Grune and Stratton (1978).
BLACK, H. C., *Black's Law Dictionary.* St. Paul, Minn.: West Publishing Company (1968).
LEHRHOFF, I., and KORASHEC, S., *Speech and Language Procedure Manual.* Beverly Hills, Calif.: Irwin Lehrhoff and Associates (no date).
NICHOLAS, T., *How to Form Your Own Corporation Without a Lawyer for Under $50.00.* Wilmington, Dela.: Enterprise Publishing Company (1977).
You and the Law (2nd Revised Ed.). Pleasantville, N.Y.: Reader's Digest Association (1977).

10

Legal and Ethical Considerations in Clinical Research

Almost all of the research conducted by speech-language pathologists and audiologists involves the use of human subjects. There has been considerable interest since the Nuremberg trials (which were conducted after World War II) in the mental and physical welfare of persons who serve as subjects in research studies. This interest has resulted in the creation of regulations on both national and international levels (see Appendix B) that are intended to protect the rights of such persons. It also has stimulated considerable discussion about ethical aspects of how human subjects are used in clinical research (see, e.g., Freund, 1970).

Some of the legal and ethical considerations in designing *clinical* research (particularly therapy outcome research) in speech-language pathology and audiology are indicated in this chapter. Most of these considerations also apply to the design of *basic* research studies in which human subjects are used.

NEED FOR PROTECTING RESEARCH SUBJECTS

Many institutions (including hospitals, universities, and school systems) have established committees that are supposed to scrutinize the design of all research projects using as subjects persons being served by the institution for possible hazards to their physical or mental well-being. These committees usually have the power to refuse to allow such persons to be used in studies that they feel carry an *unacceptably high risk* of mental or physical injury. The decision of what would constitute an unacceptably high risk probably would take into consideration the *potential benefits* of the particular study, both to the subjects and to society. The subjects would almost certainly be considered in the evaluation of a proposal for a therapy outcome study.

Why are such committees needed? Those who volunteer to serve as subjects are likely to assume that they will be *protected by the experimenter* from being harmed in any way. They would be particularly likely to make this assumption if they are volunteering to participate in an experiment from which they could not expect to benefit personally. (Subjects can benefit personally by participating in an experiment in several ways, such as gaining knowledge, improving physical and/or mental health, or being paid.) They would also be particularly likely to make this assumption if the research was being conducted under the auspices of a respected institution (such as a university or hospital).

While subjects may assume that there is no possibility of their being harmed by participating in an experiment, such an assumption would not be valid. It is impossible to design an experiment that is entirely risk-free. For example, a subject could fall and injure herself as she enters the room in which the experiment is being conducted: If she had not volunteered to serve as a subject, she probably would not have been entering the room at that moment and hence would not have fallen.

Although it would be unrealistic for subjects to assume that their participation in an experiment is entirely risk-free, they could reasonably assume that the risk of being harmed is almost nonexistent if they are not informed to the contrary. This would be the assumption of our hypothetical reasonable man. Hence, an experimenter who exposed subjects to more than extremely minimal risks of harm *without first informing them* about these risks probably would be viewed by a "reasonable man" as behaving irresponsibly. The subjects, if they were harmed, could sue both the experimenter and the institution under whose auspices the research was conducted for negligence and/or some other tort (possibly battery) with a reasonable expectation of winning and being awarded damages. This is one of the factors that motivates institutions to establish committees for evaluating research proposals.

It is important that the actual risk of harm to a subject be consistent with the subject's assumption regarding the nature of this risk. How can one insure that this will be the case? Several approaches can be used to insure that a subject's *consent* to participate in an experiment is *informed*. One would be to rely on the *experimenter* both to minimize risks to subjects and to inform them voluntarily about the risks remaining. While this would be the simplest (and probably the most common) approach, it has several limitations. Perhaps its main limitation is that the goals of collecting desired data and of protecting the persons from whom these data are being collected may not be compatible. Ordinarily an experimenter's primary objective is to gather the data needed to answer specific questions or to test specific hypotheses. While few experimenters would knowingly expose their subjects to highly dangerous experimental conditions without informing them about the risks, they might be tempted to be less forthright when the risks associated with experimental conditions have not been demonstrated empirically. Experimenters may hesitate to inform potential subjects about such a risk because it may discourage many of them from volunteering, thus making it impossible to undertake or complete the study. Experimenters may be able to convince themselves in such an instance that the potential benefits from the study to "society" and to themselves (e.g., for meeting promotion and tenure requirements) far outweigh the potential risks to individual subjects; since the study cannot be completed without an adequate number of subjects, they would be justified in not informing subjects about a potential risk that had not been conclusively demonstrated to exist.

A second approach that can be used for insuring that a subject's consent to participate is informed and that potential risks have been minimized and are within acceptable limits is to require the designs of all research studies that wish to use institutional clients as subjects to be scrutinized by an *institutional committee*. The mission of this committee would be to identify potential risks and to determine both whether they are within acceptable limits and whether subjects will be fully informed about them. This approach has been adopted by many institutions, including school systems, universities, and hospitals. Requiring such a committee to approve the design for a study can protect subjects in several ways. First, it would probably motivate the experimenter to design the study so as to minimize the risks to subjects and thus maximize the odds of the proposal's being approved by the committee. Also, the experimenter would hesitate to propose a study that would expose subjects to unacceptably high risks of harm because doing so could damage his or her professional reputation. Second, such a committee provides a mechanism for monitoring the degree to which subjects are informed about potential hazards and hence the degree to which their consent constitutes *informed consent*. Institutional committees may require experimenters to submit to them copies of the consent forms that subjects will be asked to sign. The committee would then decide whether the presentation of possible hazards on them is sufficiently complete and accurate for a subject's consent to constitute fully informed consent. If a subject is not fully informed about potential hazards before signing a consent form, his or her consent probably would not be recognized by a court (Fried, 1974). The concept of informed consent is dealt with in-depth elsewhere in this chapter.

While the second approach (using institutional committees) tends to be superior to the first (relying solely on the experimenter) for protecting the rights of subjects, it is not perfect. One of its limitations is that committee members may not be familiar with the methodology an investigator proposes to use and, hence, they may fail to recognize potential hazards to subjects. It is even conceivable that no committee members will be familiar with the methodology outlined in a proposal.

INFORMED CONSENT AS A VEHICLE FOR PROTECTING INVESTIGATORS AND INSTITUTIONS FROM TORT LITIGATION

Clinical research in the previous section was viewed from the perspective of the need for protecting the rights of research subjects. In this section it will be viewed from a different perspective—that of the need for protecting the rights of investigators and the institutions under whose auspices they are doing their research. If our legal system did not protect these rights, little (if any) clinical research would be undertaken, which would have an obvious detrimental impact on the health of persons in our society.

A subject's *informed consent* to participate in a study can provide the investigator and the institution under whose auspices the research was conducted with some protection against *tort litigation* arising from allegations that he or she was physically or mentally harmed by participating in the study. If a subject were aware of a particular risk associated with participating in a study before consenting to participate in it and if he were harmed in a manner predictable from this risk, he would be unlikely to be successful if he sued either the investigator or the institution.

One of the main types of torts against which a subject's informed consent to participate in a study can provide some protection is *battery*. According to Fried:

> The central concept of battery is the offense to personal dignity that occurs when another impinges on one's bodily integrity without full and valid consent. A punch in the stomach or being doused with a pail of water are classic examples. It is not necessary to show that one has been physically injured, much less that one has suffered financial loss. The injury is to dignity. That being the case, law suits have been brought and won against doctors who performed needed and successful operations, but without the consent of their patients. (1974, p. 15)

Hence, experimenting on people without their "full and valid consent" can result in litigation for battery even if they were not physically injured and even if they did not suffer financial loss. Such litigation also can result from subjecting clients to *therapy programs* without their "full and valid consent." For further information about torts, including battery, see Chapter 6.

The requirement that must be satisfied to justify intentionally invading another's bodily integrity is securing his or her *free and informed* consent to do so. According to Fried:

> To be effective the consent must be to the particular contact with the person in question, and if procured by "fraud or mistake as to the essential character" of the conduct it is invalid. . . . And it is not just active fraud or concealment which destroys consent. The doctor [or experimenter] who obtains consent has the duty to give the facts the patient [or subject] needs to make an informed choice. . . . He must tell the patient [or subject] about the benefits and risks of the treatment [or experimental condition(s)], and

how likely they are. And some courts have said that the patient must also be told about the hazards and advantages of alternative forms of treatment. (1974, pp. 19-20)

Hence, for consent to participate in an experiment to be regarded by a court as having been *free and informed*, the experimenter would have to be able to prove that subjects were not coerced into giving it and that they had been fully informed about the risks involved before they gave it.

Under some circumstances a subject's free and informed consent to participate in a study *may* not be essential. One such circumstance would be when the subject is a *child*, particularly a very young child who would be unable to understand the experimenter's explanation of the risks and benefits from participating in the study and hence would be incapable of giving informed consent. Consent in such a circumstance would have to be obtained from the child's legal guardian, who in most instances would be a parent. However, a guardian's ability to consent to a child's serving as a research subject is limited: "The tendency of the law has been to limit what may be done to children and incompetents just because they are unable to give effective consent. And those who act for them are strictly charged to act only in the manifest interests of these persons. They may not, for instance, volunteer them for experimentation which will *not directly* [italics mine] benefit them" (Fried, 1974, p. 23). The message here appears to be that securing a guardian's consent for his or her child to serve as a subject may not be adequate to protect against tort litigation either the experimenter or the institution under whose auspices the research is being conducted.

A subject's free and informed consent also may not be essential if he or she is an adult whom the court would classify as *incompetent*. Adults are likely to be classified as incompetent if they are thought to be unable to make rational decisions regarding their own welfare. Persons diagnosed as psychotic or severely mentally retarded are likely to be classified as incompetent. Persons who are *severely communicatively handicapped* (e.g., global aphasics) also may be classified as incompetent. A court-appointed guardian could consent to such a person's serving as a subject: The restrictions on the guardian's ability to do so are the same as were given for guardians of children.

A subject can *withdraw* consent to participate in a study at any time, even if the subject promised when giving consent not to withdraw it (Fried, 1974). The 1971 National Institute of Health policy statement on the protection of human subjects, in fact, not only mandates that subjects be allowed to withdraw consent at any time but requires that subjects *be informed* that they have this right.

LEGAL-ETHICAL IMPLICATIONS OF THE THERAPEUTIC-NONTHERAPEUTIC CONTINUUM IN CLINICAL RESEARCH

The legal doctrines that apply to a particular clinical study are determined in part by whether the experimental conditions administered to subjects are intended to be therapeutic to them. Some studies are *entirely therapeutic* in their intent. An example would be an investigation conducted by a speech-language pathologist of the impacts of a certain therapy program on the clients in it. The assumption is being made that the clinician would have used this therapy program with these clients even if its impact was not being investigated. A clinician functioning in this dual role could be labeled a clinician-investigator (Silverman, 1977).

At the other end of the continuum would be studies in which the investigator had *no therapeutic intent.* The subjects in such studies would be unlikely to benefit personally from participating in them. They may, however, be providing data that could contribute to improving therapy programs for others with similar communicative disorders at some future date. An example would be an investigation by an audiologist of the responses of persons having a particular type of lesion in the auditory system to a particular type of auditory test. The audiologist's intent is to use the subjects' responses to the test stimuli to refine the test rather than to benefit subjects directly.

There are clinical studies that fall on the continuum between these extremes. In these studies some of the experimental conditions have a therapeutic intent and others do not. Or the experimental conditions are intended to be therapeutic for some subjects but not for others. An example of the first would be a study in which clients are given one or more diagnostic tests in addition to those they would ordinarily be given for clinical purposes. Those that ordinarily would be administered for clinical purposes constitute experimental conditions having a therapeutic intent; the others constitute experimental conditions that are not intended to be therapeutic.

An example of a clinical study in which the experimental conditions are intended to be therapeutic for some subjects but not for others would be a study in which subjects are *randomly assigned* to one of two treatment groups. The subjects assigned to the first group (the experimental group) would be administered a treatment (experimental condition) that was intended to be therapeutic and hence could directly benefit them. Those assigned to the second group (the control group) either would be administered no treatment or would be administered a treatment that the experimenter did not expect to be as successful as the one administered to subjects in the first group. Thus, the subjects in the first group either would be expected to benefit directly, and those in the second group either would not be expected to benefit directly or would not be expected to benefit to the same extent as those in the first group.

Nontherapeutic Clinical Research

While persons who function as subjects in nontherapeutic clinical research may receive a small sum of money and/or personal satisfaction for doing so, they are unlikely to benefit directly in any substantial way from the experience. And by participating in the research they are risking their mental and/or physical health. In some types of research the risks to their health would be almost nonexistent; in others the risks would be substantial.

It has been argued (Fried, 1974) that there are no special legal doctrines that apply to nontherapeutic clinical research and that those that do apply (particularly with regard to the need for disclosing potential hazards) are the same as those that apply to the selling of products:

> *In general, the law imposes a strict duty of disclosure, wherever an individual with a great deal to lose is exposed to a risk or is asked to relinquish rights by someone with considerably greater knowledge* [italics mine]. And this is true, whether the relation is one of buyer and seller or involves some public interest. Persons selling cosmetics, automobiles, or pharmaceuticals are required to make full disclosure of all the hazards involved in the products they sell. . . . There is no reason why the case should be any different where a researcher asks an experimental subject to risk his health. (Fried, 1974, p. 27)

Since experimenters would ordinarily have considerably greater knowledge of the potential risks associated with the methodology being used than would their subjects and since their subjects are risking their health by participating in the experiment, experimenters are obliged to make a full disclosure of potential hazards to subjects when seeking their consent to participate. It could be argued that the failure of the experimenter to do so would be more damaging with this type of research if a subject sued for battery than it would be with research having a therapeutic intent.

While it is almost always desirable to be able to document a subject's informed consent to participate in research, there are some types of nontherapeutic studies for which failure to do so ordinarily would result in minimal risks to either investigators or the institutions under whose auspices their research is being conducted. These are studies that involve only slight or remote risks of harm to subjects. The U.S. Department of Health and Human Services, for example, in its *Final Regulations Amending Basic HHS Policy for the Protection of Human Research Subjects (Federal Register,* January 26, 1981) classified the following types of research as involving no, slight, or only remote risks of harm to subjects:

1. Research conducted in established or commonly accepted educational settings, involving normal educational practices, such as (i) research on regular and special education instructional strategies, or (ii) research on the effectiveness of or the comparison among instructional techniques, curricula, or classroom management methods.
2. Research involving the use of educational tests (cognitive, diagnostic, aptitude, achievement), if information taken from these sources are recorded in such a manner that subjects cannot be identified, directly or through identifiers linked to the subjects.
3. Research involving survey or interview procedures, except where all of the following conditions exist: (i) responses are recorded in such a manner that the human subjects can be identified, directly or through identifiers linked to the subjects, (ii) the subject's responses, if they became known outside the research, could reasonably place the subject at risk of criminal or civil liability or be damaging to the subject's financial standing or employability, and (iii) the research deals with sensitive aspects of the subject's own behavior, such as illegal conduct, drug use, sexual behavior, or use of alcohol. . . .

Research involving the observation (including the observation by participants) of public behavior, except where all of the following conditions exist: (i) observations are recorded in such a manner that the human subjects can be identified, directly or through identifiers linked to the subjects, (ii) the observations recorded about the individual, if they become known outside the research, could reasonably place the subject at risk of criminal or civil liability or be damaging to the subject's financial standing or employability, and (iii) the research deals with sensitive aspects of the subject's own behavior such as illegal conduct, drug use, sexual behavior, or use of alcohol.

4. Research involving the collection or study of existing data, documents, pathological specimens, or diagnostic specimens, if these sources are publicly available or if the information is recorded by the investigator in such a manner that subjects cannot be identified, directly or through identifiers linked to the subjects. (*Federal Register,* January 26, 1981, pp. 8371-8372)

How would a person be compensated for harm resulting from his or her participation (as a subject) in a nontherapeutic research study? Such a person probably would have to initiate some type of tort litigation against the investigator and/or the institution under whose auspices the research was being conducted. A number of authorities on legal-ethical implications of using human subjects in research (e.g., Fried, 1974; Ladimer, 1970) have stated that investigators and their institutions have a moral obligation to voluntarily compensate subjects harmed in nontherapeutic research. Perhaps a special liability insurance could be carried by investigators or their institutions for this purpose.

For further information about legal-ethical aspects of nontherapeutic clinical research, see Freund (1970), Fried (1974), and *IRB: A Review of Human Subjects Research* (a newsletter published by the Hastings Center, Institute of Society, Ethics, and the Life Sciences, 360 Broadway, Hastings-on-Hudson, New York 10706).

Therapeutic Clinical Research

Speech-language pathologists, audiologists, and other clinicians legally are justified only in using accepted therapies unless their clients specifically consent to the use of an experimental therapy. An *accepted therapy,* in this context, is a treatment program that at least some of one's professional peers would regard as appropriate for the particular condition being treated. If a speech-language pathologist treated a stutterer with a therapy program that at least some authorities on stuttering would regard as appropriate, this program would be likely to be classified as *accepted* therapy by the courts. It would not be necessary that all authorities on stuttering regard it as appropriate. The courts recognize that there are often different "schools of thought" on the appropriate therapy for a condition and, hence, they will classify as accepted almost any therapy advocated by a recognized authority.

So long as the therapy program being used in the research is one that would be classified by the courts as accepted, the legal-ethical considerations (e.g., informed consent) would be essentially the same as for *clinical treatment.*

The further away an experimental therapy program lies from the standard and the accepted, the more acute the need for subjects to be fully informed about risks and *alternative treatment programs,* and the greater the need for the investigator to be able to document the subjects' free and informed consent to participate in research. The investigator's obligation to inform subjects about alternative treatment programs ordinarily does not extend to other alternative programs (Fried, 1974). The information presented about the experimental program should include a statement summarizing research findings and professional opinion relevant to its efficacy.

A situation that may pose a legal-ethical dilemma for an investigator is one in which there are alternative treatment programs that are regarded by other professionals as *effective* for treating the condition the experimental program is intended to treat. Full disclosure requires that the subjects be informed about these alternatives. However, informing potential subjects about such alternatives may cause them to refuse to participate in the experimental program. An investigator may be tempted, therefore, to make a less than full disclosure about alternative treatment programs in order to insure having an adequate number of subjects for the research. While doing so may increase the probability of having an adequate number of subjects for the research, it also could invalidate the subjects' consent to participate in the research, leaving the investigator vulnerable to several types of tort litigation, including battery. An investigator when confronted with this situation would be wise to make a full disclosure, including a statement summarizing research and professional opinion relevant to why the experimental therapy *may* be superior to existing accepted alternative treatment programs. An investigator should be able to develop such a statement—otherwise, one could reasonably question whether it would be *ethical* to expose subjects to an experimental treatment program that there is no reason to believe is superior to existing accepted ones. Institutional research committees have a responsibility to determine whether proposed experimental treatment programs have a reasonable chance of satisfying a *real need.*

Mixed Therapeutic and Nontherapeutic Clinical Research

The type of clinical research that tends to have the greatest legal-ethical perplexities associated with it is that which has both therapeutic and nontherapeutic aspects. A speech-language pathologist or audiologist, for example, who was engaged in therapy outcome research would indeed be attempting to ameliorate the client's communicative disorder (which would be the *therapeutic aspect*). The intervention strategy chosen, however, would not be selected *solely* from the perspective of the client's needs. Therapy would be administered in the context of a research program that was intended either to test new procedures or to compare the efficacy of various established procedures (which would be the *nontherapeutic aspect*).

Hence, the treatment that a client received would be dictated, at least partially, by the requirements of the research design. In a study of the relative efficacy of two established procedures, the one the client is administered is likely to be determined by a table of random numbers. And in a study of the efficacy of a new procedure (experimental therapy), the decision whether a particular subject would be given it would be partially a function of the investigator's need for subjects with particular *demographic characteristics* (e.g., age and sex) to meet the requirements of the research design.

If the treatment dictated by a research design is the one that a client would have received anyway, then the presence of a research design ordinarily would not create any special legal-ethical problems. However, if the treatment dictated by a research design is *not* the one that a client ordinarily would have received, then the presence of a research design could create legal-ethical problems.

In clinical research having both therapeutic and nontherapeutic aspects, there obviously is a legal obligation to make a full disclosure of *possible benefits and hazards.* This would be necessary even if the therapy that the clients were receiving was not part of a research project. Would it also be necessary to disclose (1) that at least some of the therapy they will be receiving *is part of a research project* and (2) the *nature* of the research project and the experimental design? A speech-language pathologist who was planning to describe the therapy program used with a client in an individual case study in an article published in a professional journal (e.g., *Journal of Speech and Hearing Disorders*) would have to answer that question. Would the client's consent be needed to publish the case study? If it were *impossible* for anyone to recognize the client from the information included in the case study, the answer to this question probably would be *no.* A client may be recognizable not only from a name or initials but also from specific information about his or her life history, such as the names of schools attended. An investigator would be wise, therefore, to carefully examine the life history data on subjects of case studies and to delete any nonessential information that could make them recognizable. Of course, the client (or the client's guardian) in some instances would be very willing to have a description of the therapy received published, particularly if (1) the client felt treatment was successful and/or (2) the client was convinced that the information presented could help in the treatment of others with similar conditions.

While clinicians who do not disclose to a client that the therapy is part of a research project or who do not describe the *impact* that being part of a research project will have on the therapy the client will be receiving may be relatively safe legally, they may find themselves vulnerable from a *public relations* perspective. Most clients, for example, probably would feel that they had been deceived if they discovered they received the therapy program they did because they were assigned to a particular treatment group by a table of random numbers. Such a discovery could adversely affect the client-clinician relationship if they were still in therapy. And the disclosure of such a discovery in the media could severely damage the reputation both of the investigator and the institution under whose auspices the re-

RESPONSIBLE INVESTIGATOR:

TITLE OF PROTOCOL:

TITLE OF CONSENT FORM *(if different from protocol):*

I have been asked to participate in a research study that is investigating *(describe purpose of study).* In participating in this study I agree to *(describe briefly and in lay terms procedures to which subject is consenting).*

I understand that

a) The possible risks of this procedure include *(list known risks or side effects; if none, so state).* Alternative treatments include *(list alternative treatments and briefly describe advantages and disadvantages of each; if none, so state).*

b) The possible benefits of this study to me are *(enumerate; if none, so state).*

c) Any questions I have concerning my participation in this study will be answered by *(list names and degrees of people who will be available to answer questions).*

d) I may withdraw from the study at any time without prejudice.

e) The results of this study may be published, but my name or identity will not be revealed and my records will remain confidential unless disclosure of my identity is required by law.

f) My consent is given voluntarily without being coerced or forced.

g) In the event of physical injury resulting from the study, medical care and treatment will be available at this institution.

For eligible veterans, compensation (damages) may be payable under 38USC 351 or, in some circumstances, under the Federal Tort claims Act.

For non-eligible veterans and non-veterans, compensation would be limited to situations where negligence occurred and would be controlled by the provisions of the Federal Tort Claims Act.

For clarification of these laws, contact the District Counsel (213) 824-7379.

_____   _____
DATE   PATIENT OR RESPONSIBLE PARTY

                         _____
                         PATIENT'S SOCIAL SECURITY NUMBER

                         _____
                         AUDITOR/WITNESS

                         _____
                         INVESTIGATOR/PHYSICIAN REPRESENTATIVE

FIGURE 10-1 Outline for a consent form for documenting a person's informed consent to serve as a subject in a research project. (From Purtile, R. D., and Cassel, C. K., Ethical Dimensions in the Health Professions. Philadelphia: W. B. Saunders (1981).

search was conducted. The general public would tend to regard the random assignment of subjects to treatment groups without their knowledge as irresponsible, even if the therapy subjects received had been successful.

DOCUMENTING A PERSON'S INFORMED CONSENT TO SERVE AS A RESEARCH SUBJECT

An outline of a form for documenting a person's informed consent to serve as a subject in a research project is presented in Figure 10-1. This outline includes the information that ordinarily is necessary for explaining to potential subjects (1) the purpose and value of the study, (2) what they will be asked to do and what will be done to them, and (3) the possible benefits and risks to them. It also provides a means for documenting that subjects were informed that they may withdraw their consent at any time and that they have consented to having information about them published (if they cannot be recognized). In addition, it provides documentation that their consent was given freely (that it was not coerced or forced). Paragraph *g* in Figure 10-1 would be included only if provision had been made for compensating subjects for injuries that they receive (e.g., if the investigator or the institution had liability insurance that covered such injuries). Note that subjects' signatures should be witnessed. Obviously, if the information presented in the form was inaccurate or incomplete, a subject's signature on it might not constitute *informed* consent. Whether it would constitute informed consent would depend on how essential the inaccurate or incomplete information was for alerting subjects to potential risks.

REFERENCES

Final regulations amending basic HHS policy for the protection of human research subjects. *Federal Register,* 46, 8366-8392 (1981).

FREUND, P. (Ed.), *Experimentation with Human Subjects.* New York: George Braziller (1970).

FRIED, C., *Medical Experimentation: Personal Integrity and Social Policy.* New York: American Elsevier (1974).

LADIMER, I., Protection and compensation for injury in human studies. In Paul A. Freund (Ed.), *Experimentation with Human Subjects.* New York: George Braziller (1970).

PURTILO, R. B., and CASSEL, C. K., *Ethical Dimensions in the Health Professions.* Philadelphia: W. B. Saunders (1981).

SILVERMAN, F. H., *Research Design in Speech Pathology and Audiology.* Englewood Cliffs, N.J.: Prentice-Hall (1977).

11

Serving as an Expert Witness

A speech-language pathologist or audiologist can be asked to testify as a *fact* or *expert* witness at a civil or criminal court proceeding or at a hearing. The hearing probably would be conducted under the auspices of an administrative agency such as a state department of education or a local school board. An example would be a due-process hearing convened by a local school board to comply with certain requirements of Public Law 94-142 (see Appendix C).

A *fact witness* "testifies to what he has seen, heard, or otherwise observed" (Black, 1968, p. 1778). An audiologist might be asked to testify about the hearing of a person who he had tested. Or a speech-language pathologist might be asked to testify about the therapy she administered to a client. Fact witnesses testify about events they have observed—their role ordinarily is to provide rather than evaluate evidence. Their only special qualifications are that they were present when an event took place and they are willing to describe what they observed.

Expert witnesses, on the other hand, both provide and evaluate evidence. Their special qualifications are that they possess "peculiar knowledge, wisdom, skill, or information regarding subject matter under consideration, acquired by study, investigation, observation, practice or experience and not likely to be possessed by ordinary layman or inexperienced person" (Black, 1968, p. 688) and that they have "acquired ability to deduce correct inferences from hypothetical stated facts, or from facts involving scientific or technical knowledge" (Black, 1968, p. 688). They can assist the judge, the jury, and the attorney who retains them in performing their functions, particularly with regard to dealing with subject matter that requires more than a lay-person's knowledge to evaluate and/or comprehend.

Expert witnesses may or may not appear in court. If they *will not* appear in court, they function as *consultants* to the attorneys who retain them. An expert witness's remarks, conclusions, and opinions ordinarily are protected—they need not be exposed to the opposing attorney. Of course, the attorney who retains the expert can expose these remarks to the opposing attorney if he or she feels that doing so would be advantageous to the client (e.g., to encourage the other party to drop the suit or to accept an out-of-court settlement).

When expert witnesses appear in court, their remarks, conclusions, and opinions ordinarily are not protected and will be *carefully* scrutinized by the opposing attorney. The opposition will attempt to reduce the positive impact of the experts' testimony on the judge and jury by casting doubt on their credibility as experts and/or the validity of their conclusions and opinions through *cross-examination*. The attorney who retains the expert witness will attempt to establish the expert's credibility and the validity of his or her testimony sufficiently strongly so that even after cross-examination the expert testimony will have the desired impact on the judge and jury.

SUBJECTS ABOUT WHICH SPEECH-LANGUAGE PATHOLOGISTS AND AUDIOLOGISTS HAVE TESTIFIED AS EXPERT WITNESSES

Expert witnesses function in both civil and criminal court proceedings and in hearings. Speech-language pathologists and audiologists have testified as experts in all three types of proceedings. Some of the subjects about which they have been asked to testify are indicated in this section.

Criminal Court Proceedings

In criminal cases speech-language pathologists and audiologists have probably most often been asked to provide expert testimony (1) to establish the *competency* of a defendant to be tried and (2) to confirm the *identification* of a defendant through his or her speech or voice.

Under our legal system, a person ordinarily cannot be tried and convicted for committing a crime unless he or she is judged *legally competent*. An aspect of being legally competent is being able to comprehend what is transpiring during the trial. "In the United States of America it is a firmly established principle of law that a person cannot be put on trial if his condition is such that he will not be able to understand the proceedings and make a proper defense" (Meyers, 1968, p. 130). This would ordinarily be the case for a person who is deaf, and unable to speak, and unable to comprehend sign language or any other language system. It also could be the case for a severe receptive or global aphasic. The role of the expert witness in such an instance would be to assess the communicative competency of the defendant and to testify about it to the court.

The prosecution has introduced as evidence in some criminal cases an *identification of a defendant* based on the person's speech or voice. A prosecutor may wish to introduce such evidence to prove, for example, that a defendant made certain obscene telephone calls. In such cases the prosecutor may attempt to introduce as evidence an acoustic analysis of a recorded speech sample known as a *voice print* (Block, 1975). The identification of persons from their speech or voice patterns is controversial, and speech-language pathologists have been asked to testify as expert witnesses both supporting (for the prosecution) and questioning (for the defense) the validity and reliability of such identification.

Civil Court Proceedings

In civil cases speech-language pathologists and audiologists have most often been asked to provide expert testimony on (1) competency, (2) personal injury, and (3) custody of minors in divorce cases (Fox, 1978).

Speech-language pathologists and audiologists have been asked to testify about a person's *competency* in civil as well as criminal court proceedings. In a civil case they would testify about a person's competency to manage his or her financial and other affairs rather than competency to stand trial. Some members of an aphasic's family, for example, may seek to have him declared incompetent to manage his affairs (Rada, Porch, and Kellner, 1975). A speech-language pathologist could be asked to testify as an expert in such an instance by the attorney representing either the family or the aphasic.

In *personal injury* cases the court must establish the extent of the injury and the prognosis for improvement before it can determine how much compensation the injured party should be awarded. Such cases include proceedings for malpractice (see Chapter 6) and worker's compensation. Speech-language pathologists and audiologists have been asked to examine a plaintiff's speech, language, or hearing and to testify as an expert about the extent to which a communicative disorder is handicapping to the plaintiff and the likelihood that the degree of handicap will be lessened in the future. An audiologist, for example, may be asked to testify as an expert about the hearing of a person who is seeking *worker's compensation* for a hearing loss that she claims resulted from exposure to high levels of noise at her place of employment. Or a speech-language pathologist may be asked to testify as an expert about the aphonia of a person who is suing an anesthetist for *malpractice* because he claims that the anesthetist damaged his vocal folds when he passed a tube between them during a surgical procedure.

A speech-language pathologist or audiologist may be asked to testify as an expert in cases concerned with the *custody of minors in divorce cases*. Family courts are supposed to award custody of minor children to the parent who can best meet their needs. If a child has a communicative disorder that requires treatment, one factor the court probably will consider when deciding on custody is the ability of each parent to make it possible for the child to receive necessary therapy. If one parent planned to reside in a rural area where therapy would not be readily available and the other planned to reside in an urban area where it would be readily available, the court (at least with regard to this factor) would tend to favor the "urban" rather than the "rural" parent. In custody cases speech-language pathologists and audiologists would ordinarily testify about such matters as the therapy and special educational needs of the child and the likelihood of being able to meet these needs where each parent plans to reside. They might also testify about the ability of each parent to cope with problems arising from the child's communicative disorder. One parent, for example, might be able to understand almost all of the child's speech, and the other to understand little of it.

Administrative Agency Hearings

Administrative agencies conduct hearings that are somewhat similar in format to court proceedings. In fact, they are sometimes referred to as *quasi-judicial* proceedings. One feature they share with court proceedings is the use of expert witnesses and consultants. A speech-language pathologist or audiologist is probably more likely to be asked to testify as an expert at the hearing than at a civil or criminal court proceeding.

Speech-language pathologists and audiologists are frequently asked to testify as experts at hearings associated with Public Law 94-142, which mandates local school districts to meet the special educational needs of all children residing in the geographical area they serve. If the parents of a child feel that their school district is not adequately meeting the child's needs, they can request a hearing at which they would probably be represented by an attorney. Assuming the child has a communicative disorder, the attorney retained by the parents may ask a speech-language pathologist or audiologist to examine the child and testify as an expert about the child's special educational needs and the services required. Or the attorney representing the school district may make such a request in an attempt to establish that it is adequately meeting the child's needs.

FUNCTIONING AS AN EXPERT WITNESS

This section presents some guidelines for functioning as an expert witness in a court proceeding or hearing. They were synthesized from several sources intended for preparing physicians to serve as expert witnesses. The order in which they are presented is not necessarily related to their importance. They are intended to supplement rather than substitute for a pretrial (or prehearing) conference with the attorney requesting the services.

Projecting an Appropriate Image

The impact that an expert's testimony has on a judge and jury is determined not only by what he or she says, but also by his or her conduct while testifying. If they perceive the expert as someone who is both *knowledgeable* about the subject and *confident* about the accuracy of the testimony, they will tend to give the testimony more weight than they will if they feel that he or she is not knowledgeable about the subject or not confident about the accuracy of some of his or her testimony. Also, if the expert does not *dress appropriately* (i.e., in a manner consistent with expectations of how an "expert" should dress) or *communicate well,* his or her testimony may be given less credibility than it deserves. While it is unfortunate that the manner in which experts conduct themselves can profoundly influence the impact of their testimony on a judge and jury, it is nevertheless a fact of life with which expert witnesses must contend. Hence, those testifying as experts must seek to conduct themselves in a manner that will maximize the probability that the judge and jury will give appropriate weight to their testimony.

Any number of variables can influence the image that an expert witness projects, including the following:

1. The amount of *eye contact* the expert has with the judge and jury (particularly the latter). Having frequent eye contact with them while testifying ordinarily will enhance a witness's image.

2. The extent to which the expert can maintain his or her *composure.* The more successful the expert witness is at reflecting confidence and assurance while testifying, the more credence the judge and jury will give to the testimony. Hence, during cross-examination the opposing attorney is likely to attempt to get the expert to lose his or her composure.

3. The extent to which the witness establishes his or her *qualifications* to testify as an expert. The more successful he or she is at establishing these qualifications, the more credible the judge and jury will tend to regard the testimony. The opposing attorney may attempt to nullify the testimony by questioning the witness's qualifications to testify as an expert about the matter at hand.

4. The extent to which the witness succeeds at *communicating* with the judge and jury. Some experts attempt to impress a jury by using many esoteric scientific terms. This is a questionable strategy. A jury is more likely to be persuaded by an expert who attempts to communicate with them in language they can understand. An expert witness should assume that the members of the jury know nothing about his or her field of expertise and take on a responsibility to communicate findings and opinions to them in language they can understand. Obviously, while doing this an expert should be careful not to appear to be talking down to them.

5. The extent to which the expert has *reviewed the testimony* with the attorney who retained him or her. If the attorney either is unaware of or does not understand what the expert can say that may be helpful to the client, the attorney may not ask the appropriate questions during *direct examination.* An expert ordinarily testifies during direct examination by answering a series of questions asked by the attorney who retained him or her. If all the questions that need to be answered in order to present the testimony are not asked, then the expert's testimony may not have the positive impact on the judge and jury that it deserves. The attorney may ask the expert to formulate a series of questions, the answers to

which would allow the testimony to be presented in a relatively complete, clear, and organized manner.

A *second reason* why the expert should review the testimony with the attorney is to indicate how the opposing attorney may seek to refute the testimony during cross-examination. If the attorney is aware of this, he or she will probably be better prepared to deal with the negative impact of cross-examination on the expert's testimony by asking the expert appropriate questions during *redirect examination*.

A *third reason* why the expert should meet with the attorney prior to appearing in court is to make certain that the attorney knows enough about the expert's background to convince the judge and jury that he or she is qualified to testify as an expert about the matter at hand. The attorney, to establish the credibility of the expert, asks a series of questions at the *beginning* of the direct examination. (A representative set of such questions is presented elsewhere in this chapter.) The expert witness can be helpful to the attorney by reviewing these questions to make certain they will allow the expert witness to present the information necessary to establish credibility as an expert.

6. The *directness* with which the expert witness answers questions. If an expert is perceived by the judge and jury as being *evasive* or *defensive* when answering questions, the potential positive impact of the testimony on the judge and jury is likely to be reduced. An expert witness must be particularly careful not to appear evasive when asked by the opposing attorney (during cross-examination) to answer yes or no to a question that the expert believes cannot be adequately answered with a simple yes or no. In such a situation an expert witness is permitted to appeal to the judge. The judge may allow the witness to give a fuller answer, but if not, the expert *should not argue* about it. The attorney who retained the expert can provide an opportunity to answer more fully during redirect examination.

7. The *respect* the expert shows for judge and jury. The judge is the "boss" of the court and the expert witness should always show respect. Failure to do so can adversely affect the image that the members of the jury have of the expert since they tend to expect witnesses to be respectful of the judge. It also can result in the expert's being cited by the judge for *contempt of court*.

8. Whether the jury believes that the expert is being *paid for testifying*. An expert witness ordinarily receives a fee—not for the testimony, but for the time, professional knowledge, and services for studying the facts of the case and for formulating expert opinions based on these facts. If the opposing attorney (during cross-examination) can make the jury believe that the expert testified as he or she did because of the fee received, they are apt to give little weight to the testimony.

Testifying

An expert witness's testimony ordinarily can be divided into four parts. The first part consists of answers to questions about personal background and experience, which are asked by the attorney who retained him or her. Its purpose is to establish credibility to testify as an expert about the matter at hand.

The second part consists of answers to questions about the case, which are asked by the attorney who retained him or her. These questions and answers are the "meat" of the expert's *direct testimony.*

The third part consists of answers to questions about the direct testimony, which are asked by the opposing attorney. These questions are likely to deal both with the expert's qualifications to testify as an expert about the matter at hand and with the expert's testimony about the case. This part is referred to as *cross-examination.* It is an attempt to nullify the expert's direct testimony by suggesting to the jury that he or she is not qualified to testify as an expert about the matter at hand or that his or her interpretations (opinions) are not the only possible ones.

The fourth part consists of answers to questions about the testimony during cross-examination, which are asked by the attorney who retained him or her. The attorney's objective during this part (which is referred to as the *redirect* examination) is to reestablish the qualifications of the witness and to establish that the interpretations (opinions) given in testimony are more viable than those suggested by the opposing attorney during cross-examination.

Some guidelines for testifying as an expert during each of these four parts are presented in the following paragraphs.

Being Qualified as an Expert The first task of the attorney who retained the expert witness is to establish during direct examination that the witness is competent to testify as an expert about the matter at hand. If the attorney is successful, the *trial judge will rule* that the witness is competent to testify as an expert. The attorney will then go on to the substantive part of the direct examination.

To qualify the witness as an expert, the attorney asks a series of questions. The following series, which was abstracted from several sources (Imwinkelried, 1980; Jeans, 1975; Mauet, 1980; and Moenssens, 1973) is representative:

Q: Will you state your name, please?
Q: Will you state your business address, please?
Q: What is your business occupation?
Q: What is your present title?
Q: For how long have you been employed in this occupation?
Q: Will you briefly describe, please, the subject matter of this occupation?
Q: Do you specialize within this occupation?
Q: What is your speciality?
Q: What is it concerned with?
Q: How long have you been in practice in this speciality?
Q: What is your formal education?
Q: Which undergraduate school did you attend?
Q: What degree did you obtain there?
Q: What was your major field of study?
Q: What graduate school(s) did you attend?
Q: What degree(s) did you obtain there?

Q: What was your major field of study?
Q: What postgraduate training have you received?
Q: Are you licensed (or certified) to practice this occupation?
Q: By whom was this license (or certification) awarded?
Q: For how long have you had it?
Q: What positions have you held since the completion of your formal training?
Q: For how long did you hold each?
Q: To what professional organizations do you belong?
Q: What are the qualifications for becoming a member of these organizations?
Q: What offices and committee assignments have you held in these organizations?
Q: Have you taught courses in your speciality?
Q: Where?
Q: Have you published articles or books?
Q: How many articles have you published?
Q: In what scientific journals did they appear?
Q: How many books have you published?
Q: What are the titles of these books?
Q: What topics did you discuss in these articles and books?
Q: Have you ever testified in court as an expert witness?
Q: What subjects have you testified on?
Q: How many clients who were diagnosed as having ..... have you treated?
Q: Have you ever previously evaluated a client for (e.g., competency to manage his financial affairs)?
Q: How many times have you performed such an evaluation?

The specific questions that an expert witness will be asked depend on the expert's background and experience and the subject matter about which he or she will be testifying. For example, if the expert has not published any works, this question will not be asked.

The opposing attorney is entitled to cross-examine the witness about these qualifications. He or she may do so at this stage in the proceeding or wait until the direct examination has been completed.

An expert witness should not feel compelled to answer questions immediately after they are asked; it is wise to avoid appearing either *too willing* or *reluctant*. When answering, he or she should be brief and to the point, not volunteering extra information but answering only the questions asked. If a question is not clearly phrased, the witness should not hesitate to ask the attorney to clarify it. If the attorney makes an inaccurate remark or interprets testimony in a way that is not completely accurate, the expert should make a correction; otherwise, the opposing attorney probably will.

Direct Examination After the trial judge rules that the witness is competent to testify as an expert, the attorney begins the questioning about the matter that is to be the subject of testimony. Some questions are likely to be *fact* questions about the person who has the communicative disorder and the services the person has received. Others will be *opinion* questions. The witness may be asked to give an opinion based on the *facts* (evidence) in the case or on a series of assumptions. The latter involves answering a *hypothetical question.* An answer to such a question should conform to the facts that are substantiated in the evidence of the case.

An expert witness should avoid bringing written records to court if at all possible. When records are used while testifying, they become part of the evidence. The opposing attorney can examine them, comment on them, and read from them to the judge and jury. An expert witness would be unwise, therefore, to bring any written records that he or she would not want to have read aloud in court.

Ordinarily an expert witness is permitted to use *exhibits* and *demonstrations* to clarify points that might otherwise be confusing to a jury. Exhibits can vary from anatomical diagrams (e.g., of the ear) to audiotapes or videotapes (e.g., to demonstrate the magnitude of the person's communicative disorder). Juries tend to be fascinated by demonstrations and exhibits that show the functions of the human body. The expert witness may request a blackboard if writing or drawing on it will help make certain points. When presenting exhibits and demonstrations the expert witness should face the jury and address it directly.

Cross-Examination The opposing attorney is given the opportunity to cross-examine the expert witness after the direct examination has been completed. He or she will attempt to *nullify* any positive impact that the expert's testimony has had on the jury. Several strategies can be used for this purpose. For example, the opposing attorney might attempt to prove that the witness is not qualified to testify as an expert *about the matter at hand.* If a speech-language pathologist testified as an expert about laryngeal paralysis, the opposing attorney might attempt to prove that the clinician's previous experience with cases of laryngeal paralysis had been quite limited and, hence, the validity of the opinions stated is uncertain. Merely raising questions in the minds of the jury members about the validity of certain aspects of the expert's testimony can significantly reduce (or nullify) its positive impact on them.

Another strategy that the opposing attorney can use to nullify the positive impact of an expert's testimony is to convince the *members of the jury* that the expert was paid to testify in a certain manner. The opposing attorney might ask the witness if he or she was paid to testify. If the witness answers yes, the attorney can use this to cast doubt on the impartiality of the testimony. This point was discussed in greater depth earlier in this chapter.

A third strategy an opposing attorney can use to nullify the positive impact of an expert's testimony is to convince the members of the jury that the expert's opinions are *not the only possible viable ones.* The attorney could attempt to do this in one of several ways. He or she might attempt to get the expert witness to *admit* that (1) the interpretations and opinions put forth are not the only ones that would be consistent with the evidence or that (2) the expert cannot be completely certain about the accuracy of his or her testimony. Opposing attorneys sometimes introduce into evidence the testimony of their *own expert witnesses* to contradict that of the expert witnesses whom they are cross-examining. By so doing, they convey the message to the members of the jury that *experts disagree*. Such a message, obviously, would tend to reduce any positive impact of the expert's testimony.

The expert witness and the opposing attorney are *adversaries* during cross-examination. The attorney has a single objective—to induce the expert to behave (verbally and/or nonverbally) in a manner that will reduce (or eliminate) any positive impact that his or her testimony has had on the members of the jury. And the expert witness also has a single objective—to project to the members of the jury an image that will not reduce any positive impact that his or her testimony has had on them and will possibly *enhance* it.

During cross-examination an attorney may attempt to influence a witness's behavior in various ways, including the following:

1. To cause the witness to become angry and counterattack. If the attorney is successful, the members of the jury are likely to perceive the witness as being *less dignified* than they originally thought, which could reduce the weight that they gave to his or her testimony.
2. To cause the witness to lower his or her guard by behaving in a friendly fashion. The opposing attorney behaves in a manner that the witness interprets as *relaxed and friendly*. This is designed to cause the witness to lower any defenses and say things that will weaken the testimony. When the opposing attorney comes on in this fashion, the expert witness should *raise* rather than lower his or her guard.
3. To intimidate the witness. A cross-examiner might grimly shuffle a batch of papers while approaching the witness stand to frighten the witness into thinking that they contain evidence damaging to his or her testimony. Or the cross-examiner might write down some of the witness's responses in a very conspicuous manner, thereby suggesting that ammunition to destroy the testimony is being collected. If the attorney is successful and the witness exhibits *overt signs of fright,* not only might the expert's credibility with the members of the jury be reduced, but the expert could say things that would weaken the testimony.
4. To cause the witness to agree that an opinion may be a *speculation*. If an expert witness agrees with a cross-examiner that a particular opinion may be a speculation, the members of the jury may interpret this response to mean that the opinion is mere guess work. If a cross-examiner suggests that an opinion of an expert witness is speculation, the witness should indicate that it is not speculation but is based on *reasonable professional certainty and in accordance with scientific probability* (Sanbar, 1977).
5. To cause the witness to *disparage the expert testimony* for the opposite side. To do so could cause some members of the jury to lose respect for the witness, which could result in their giving his or her testimony less weight. If an expert witness during cross-examination is asked to explain the conflicting expert testimony for the opposite side, he or she can answer by saying, "I am sure _____ is a competent professional, but I simply do not agree on this particular issue" (Sanbar, 1977). The attorney who retained the expert witness has the responsibility for disparaging the expert testimony presented by the opposing side.

6. To cause a witness to answer a question with a yes that should be answered with a no. A cross-examiner may ask an expert witness a series of questions at a relatively rapid rate, all of which call for the answer yes and then ask one that should be answered no. Because of the rhythm the witness has developed to say yes, he or she may end up saying yes when meaning to say no.

An expert's testimony in some instances will end following cross-examination. If this is to be the case, the judge will indicate it. *An expert witness should not leave the witness stand before being told to do so by the judge.* He or she should be careful to maintain dignity when leaving the witness stand—never making any obvious victory signs or signs of relief, and not grin broadly as a sign of triumph, nor run away from the stand with unseemly haste (Sanbar, 1977).

Redirect Examination The attorney who retained the expert witness will in some instances want to ask additional questions to "repair the damage" that was done during cross-examination. The points that should be kept in mind when answering such questions are those that were mentioned in the section on direct examination.

THE EXPERT WITNESS FEE

An expert witness is ordinarily paid a fee to compensate for time and testimony-related expenses. He or she should seek to be paid an *hourly* rate rather than a lump sum fee. The hours that are compensated should include not only those spent in courts but also those incurred in making out reports, attending pretrial conferences and hearings, and gathering data (including examining the person who has the communicative disorder). The expenses should include transportation costs, hotel rooms, meals, tips, time spent on the telephone, and consultations (Sanbar, 1977). An expert witness should carefully record and, if possible, document both the amount of time spent on a case and the expenses incurred.

It is unethical for an expert witness to enter into an agreement that makes the fee *contingent* on the outcome of the trial. However, it would be ethical for him to agree to serve without guarantee of payment (Sanbar, 1977).

To avoid misunderstandings an expert witness should have a *written agreement* (contract) with the attorney who retains him or her. It should specify the amount to be paid, by whom, and when. This agreement should include a provision assuring compensation for preparations and services provided in the event that a settlement is reached before the suit is heard by a court.

REFERENCES

BLACK, C. H., *Black's Law Dictionary* (Rev. 4th Ed.). St. Paul, Minn.: West Publishing Company (1968).

BLOCK, E., *Voice Printing.* New York: David McKay (1975).
FOX, D. R., Forensic speech pathology. In R. Ray Battin and Donna R. Fox (Eds.), *Private Practice in Audiology and Speech Pathology.* New York: Grune and Stratton (1978).
IMWINKELRIED, E.J., *Evidentiary Foundations.* New York: Bobbs-Merrill (1980).
JEANS, J.W., *Trial Advocacy.* St. Paul, Minn.: West Publishing Company (1975).
MAULET, T.A., *Fundamentals of Trial Techniques.* Boston: Little, Brown and Company (1980).
MEYERS, L. J., *The Law and the Deaf.* Washington, D.C.: Vocational Rehabilitation Administration (1968).
MOENSSENS, A. A., *Scientific Evidence in Criminal Cases.* Mineola, N.Y.: Foundation Press (1973).
RADA, R. T., PORCH, B., and KELLNER, R., Aphasia and the expert medical witness. *American Academy of Psychiatry and the Law Bulletin,* 3, 231-237 (1975).
SANBAR, S. S., The expert witness. Paper presented at American Academy of Private Practice in Speech Pathology and Audiology Conference on Legal Considerations, Oklahoma City (May 1977).

12

Lobbying for Legislative Change

The 1979 Revision of the Code of Ethics of the American Speech-Language-Hearing Association (see Appendix E) requires speech-language pathologists and audiologists to "hold paramount the welfare of persons served professionally." In addition, it charges them to "expand services to persons with speech, language, and hearing problems." These injunctions imply that speech-language pathologists and audiologists have a responsibility to the communicatively handicapped that extends beyond their own caseloads, a responsibility that includes doing everything possible to insure that persons requiring speech, language, or hearing services will be able to receive them. One of the main reasons why communicatively handicapped persons may not receive needed services is *lack of funding*. The clinical services received by the *majority* of communicatively handicapped persons at this time are *not paid for directly* by them or their families. They are paid for by a *third party*, in most instances a municipal, state, or federal administrative agency. These agencies (including state departments of education and the federal Social Security Administration) are able to provide the funding because they have been allocated funds for the purpose by statutes enacted by municipal, state, or federal legislatures. Such legislatures have the ability to maintain a given level of funding for speech, language, and hearing services, to increase this level of funding, or to reduce it. The level of funding they allocate for such services is partially determined by the arguments that are presented to them for increasing, reducing, or maintaining a given level of funding. These arguments are presented to them by persons functioning as *lobbyists*.

During the 1970s the frequency with which speech-language pathologists and audiologists functioned as lobbyists for the communicatively handicapped increased considerably. This increase in activity appears to have resulted primarily from the creation of the American Speech-Language-Hearing Association's Congressional Action Contact Network. A member of the association is assigned to each member of Congress (each senator and each representative) to make the legislator aware of ASHA's position on bills that are or will be under consideration. Some state speech and hearing associations have established similar networks to inform members of their state legislatures about their position on proposed bills.

My objectives in this chapter are to facilitate in the reader the development of an "objective" attitude toward lobbying for services for the communicatively handicapped and to provide the reader with some basic information about how to function in this role. The material is presented with the hope that it will motivate some readers to participate in ASHA's Congressional Action Contact Network or comparable networks established by their state speech and hearing associations.

WHAT IS A LOBBYIST?

Any person who *consciously* attempts to influence the votes of legislators can be regarded as a lobbyist. The legislators to be influenced may be members of federal, state, or municipal legislative bodies. The lobbyist ordinarily attempts to influence them by making them aware of the position of the organization that he or she represents on a particular bill. The lobbyist may be paid by the organization or may work as a volunteer. He or she may use any of a number of approaches to influence legislators, including (1) testifying before legislative committees, (2) engaging in personal discussions with legislators to explain in detail the reasons for positions advocated, and (3) preparing briefs, memorandums, legislative analyses, and draft legislation for use by legislative committees and individual legislators. Each of these is discussed elsewhere in this chapter.

Lobbyists are granted the right to attempt to influence legislators in the *First Amendment* to the U.S. Constitution:

> Congress shall make no laws . . . abridging the freedom of speech, or of the press, or the right of the people peaceably to assemble, *and to petition the Government for a redress of grievances* [italics mine].

This right is based largely on the guarantees of free speech and the peoples' right "to petition the Government for a redress of grievances." Lobbyists have influenced the legislative process on federal, state, and municipal levels since the founding of our country (Schriftgiesser, 1951; *The Washington Lobby*, 1971).

Ethical lobbyists (as opposed to unscrupulous ones) perform an important function in the legislative process. They speak knowledgeably for various economic, commercial, minority, and other interests. Legislators are unlikely to be highly knowledgeable about the subject matter of all the bills on which they are expected to vote. To cast an informed vote on a bill, they must understand the implications of its being passed and becoming a law. Lobbyists representing *special interest groups* on both sides of a particular bill can help legislators understand its ramifications by presenting them with arguments and evidence supporting their points of view. Hence, special interest groups through their lobbyists can provide legislators with information that will allow them to cast informed votes. In a sense lobbyists advocating various positions on an issue perform a similar service for *legislators* that attorneys representing plaintiff and defendant perform in a court for the members of a *jury*—that is, presenting the strongest case that they can for their side, thereby maximizing the probability that an appropriate decision will be reached.

Most organizations (associations) have as an aspect of their mandate the encouragement of legislation consistent with the special interests shared by their members. People join an organization presumably because it allows them to interact with others who share *one* of their special interests: The organization, thereby, becomes a credible spokesperson for individuals having that special interest. It may retain a *professional* lobbyist (or lobbyists) to monitor pending legislation and, where appropriate, to present its point of view on such legislation. Or it may rely on some of its members who are not professional lobbyists to perform these functions. Or it may rely on a combination of professional lobbyists and member volunteers. (The American Speech-Language-Hearing Association uses a combination approach. The organization employs a professional lobbyist to monitor pending legislation and present its point of view to some legislators and members of their staffs. It uses member volunteers to present its point of view on pending legislation to members of the Congress when the professional lobbyist feels that doing so could be helpful.)

An organization through its lobbying activities can *indirectly* promote the welfare of its members by promoting the welfare of those who are consumers of the goods and services that its members provide. If the American Speech-Language-Hearing Association, for example, supports legislation that would provide increased services for a segment of the communicatively handicapped population, it also is encouraging an increased demand for the services provided by speech-language pathologists and audiologists and, hence, additional employment possibilities for such persons. The motivation of an organization to lobby for the welfare of those who consume the goods and/or services provided by its members, therefore, is partially altruistic and partially self-serving.

APPROACHES USED BY LOBBYISTS TO INFLUENCE LEGISLATORS

Lobbyists, both professional and volunteer, have used a variety of approaches for influencing legislators' votes. These include (1) "bribery," (2) testifying before legislative committees, (3) engaging in personal discussions with legislators to explain in detail the reasons for the positions they advocate, and (4) preparing briefs, memorandums, legislative analyses, and draft legislation for use by legislative committees and individual legislators. Some implications of each of these approaches will be indicated in this section.

"Bribery"

Bribery is one of the oldest approaches that lobbyists have used to influence legislators. In its most blatant form, it involves a payment of money (or its equivalent) to legislators in exchange for their supporting or not supporting a particular bill. The ABSCAM scandal of the early 1980s in which an FBI agent posing as a lobbyist offered bribes to a number of members of the Congress (which they accepted) for their support on a particular bill indicates that attempted bribery in its most blatant form can still occur. This approach does have a serious limitation in that it is a *crime* for a lobbyist to offer a bribe and for a legislator to accept it. A reputable organization, such as ASHA, would of course be highly unlikely to try such an approach.

The form of "bribery" in which a legislator is paid directly for a vote probably occurs relatively infrequently at this time. However, an indirect form of bribery being practiced by special interest groups appears to be quite wide-spread: Lobbyists arrange for contributions to be made to the campaign funds of certain persons running for election or reelection to a legislative body such as the U.S. Congress or a state legislature. If these persons are elected, they may feel obligated to the special interest groups who supported them, which could influence their votes on certain legislation. The potential for this form of bribery has motivated some persons to attempt to reform campaign financing (e.g., to have campaigns funded by government rather than private donations or to limit the amount that a given individual or group can contribute to a given candidate).

There is another form of "bribery" used by lobbyists that ordinarily is not regarded as being such. This includes such activities as providing legislators with meals, trips, and entertainment and inviting them to address the special interest group that the lobbyist represents. A legislator probably would receive media coverage of his or her presentation and possibly an honorarium. A state speech and hearing association that is seeking passage of a licensure bill may invite a state legislator whom they feel might be willing to sponsor the bill to be the luncheon speaker at their annual convention.

Testifying before Legislative Committees

Before a bill is considered by a particular legislative body (such as the U.S. Senate or House of Representatives), it is ordinarily considered by a *committee* made up of members of that legislative body. The mandate given to this committee is to conduct a *hearing* to explore the ramifications of the bill thoroughly. Following the hearing, the committee is expected to recommend what action the legislative body should take on the bill. Lobbyists representing special interest groups ordinarily are permitted to testify at these hearings. Their testimony consists of arguments, *supported by evidence,* indicating why the special interest group that they represent believes the bill under consideration should or should not be enacted into law. Those who testify are ordinarily questioned by members of the committee following their formal presentation. Officers of the American Speech-Language-Hearing Association and members of the National Office Staff have testified at such hearings. Officers of state speech and hearing associations and lobbyists retained by them have testified at similar hearings conducted by state legislative committees.

Personal Discussions with Legislators

The approach that is probably most effective in influencing how legislators vote is engaging in personal discussions with them about bills they are considering. This approach tends to be particularly effective when the lobbyists are *constituents* of the legislators they are attempting to influence—that is, when the lobbyist resides in the district the legislator represents. A special interest group that wished to use this approach effectively would require the services of a relatively large number of volunteer lobbyists distributed over particular geographical areas. The American Speech-Language-Hearing Association initiated its Congressional Action Contact (CAC) Network in the early 1970s to secure such a group of volunteer lobbyists. An ASHA member is selected from each congressional district (both Senate and House) to serve as the legislator's resource person (CAC) on the problems of the communicatively handicapped. CACs interact with legislators and their staffs and attempt to increase their awareness of the problems encountered by the communicatively handicapped and the implications of pending legislation on the well-being of such people. The lobbying activities of CACs are coordinated on a state level by a state coordinator and on a national level by members of the ASHA National Office Staff. Further information about the CAC network can be obtained from the ASHA National Office.

Preparing Briefs, Memorandums, Legislative Analyses, and Draft Legislation

Lobbyists often draft documents for the use of individual legislators and legislative committees. Such documents may *summarize* statistical or other data that support the point of view the lobbyist is advocating. Or they may *summarize* the organization's *position* on certain pending legislation. Or they may be *preliminary drafts of bills* that the special interest group wishes to have considered (and hopefully enacted) by a particular legislative body. A state speech and hearing association that wanted a licensure bill for speech-language pathologists and audiologists passed by its state legislature might prepare a preliminary draft of such a bill and then have the person functioning as its lobbyist attempt to locate one or more legislators who would be willing to *sponsor* it. Of course, locating a sponsor (or sponsors) does not guarantee its passage.

FUNCTIONING AS A LOBBYIST

Many speech-language pathologists and audiologists are somewhat intimidated by the thought of contacting one of their state or federal legislators and attempting to influence his or her vote on a bill. Most of us tend to view our state and federal legislators as authority figures who deal only with important issues and we assume they have little interest in the problems of the communicatively handicapped. Unfortunately, if we approach a legislator with this attitude, we are likely to communicate our anxiety. This could decrease the amount of weight that a legislator would give to our point of view. It is crucial, therefore, that when we function as lobbyists we truly believe that *what we have to say is important to the legislator.*

Lobbyists can be viewed as *behavior modifiers.* They are seeking to *shape* the behavior of a legislator. Their overall behavioral objective is to have the legislator sponsor a particular bill or vote in a particular way on it. To achieve this objective, lobbyists consciously or unconsciously use *principles of behavior modification.*

What are a lobbyist's specific behavioral objectives? One is to convince the legislator that because the position being advocated is valid, the legislator should vote in a particular way. A second objective is to convince the legislator that it would be advantageous to vote in this way. Even when legislators have been convinced that a position is valid, they may not support it if they feel that doing so could hurt them—for example, by hurting their chances for reelection.

Lobbyists apply *behavior modification principles* to achieve their behavioral objectives. They may or may not be consciously aware of doing so. By presenting arguments supported by data the lobbyist makes the legislator sympathetic to the point of view being advocated and then *positively reinforces* any comments from the legislator that suggest that his or her attitudes are changing in the direction the lobbyist desires. The lobbyist also presents arguments supported by data that are intended to convince the legislator that he or she would *gain rather than lose* by voting for (or against) a particular bill.

Information about pending legislation affecting the communicatively handicapped can be found in the *Governmental Affairs Review,* which is published quarterly by the American Speech-Language-Hearing Association. This publication reviews both federal and state legislative activity. The American Speech-Language-Hearing Association also publishes the *Congressional Action Contact Bulletin,* which includes information about bills affecting the communicatively handicapped being considered by the Congress. Information on this topic also is published in the journal *Asha.*

For further information about functioning as a volunteer lobbyist on the *national* level, contact the coordinator of the Congressional Action Contact Network at the ASHA national office. Comparable information about functioning as a volunteer lobbyist on a *state* level can be obtained from your state speech and hearing association. An informal discussion of lobbying activities for the communicatively handicapped can be found in the July 1981 issue of *Asha*.

PLAYING AN ADVOCACY ROLE

The emphasis thus far in this chapter has been on supporting the passage of bills that benefit communicatively handicapped persons. After such a bill has been passed, speech-language pathologists and audiologists have the opportunity to assume a new role in relation to it—that of an *advocate*. In this role they would do everything possible to insure that their clients receive the services they are entitled to under the law. Clients may not receive services to which they are legally entitled unless their clinicians play an advocacy role.

Why might communicatively handicapped persons not receive services to which they are legally entitled? Often they do not know about the existence of governmental programs from which they could obtain funding for needed services. Sometimes they *have been refused* services to which they are entitled by law. A state department of public instruction, for example, could refuse to fund clinical services for children who have only one or two articulation errors even though federal law (P.L. 94-142) has been interpreted to mean that they are entitled to receive such services.

The ethical responsibility mentioned earlier in this chapter to "hold paramount the welfare of persons served professionally" applies to advocacy as well as to lobbying. Holding paramount the welfare of clients implies having a responsibility to do whatever one can to make it possible for them to receive the clinical services they require. Hence, it implies a responsibility to play an advocacy role.

What would a speech-language pathologist or audiologist, as an advocate, *do for a client?* The answer to this question depends on why the client is not receiving services to which he or she is entitled. If the client was unaware of governmental programs that could provide or fund the needed services, the clinician could play an advocacy role by giving information about possible sources of funding. To do this a clinician must be aware of municipal, state, and federal programs that might fund services the client required but could not totally afford.

A speech-language pathologist or audiologist can also play an advocacy role by convincing the administrators of governmental programs that they should be providing funding for services that they are not currently funding. This assumes that the administrators are not interpreting their regulations to mean that certain services required by communicatively handicapped persons are covered and, hence, fundable. The administrators of such a program may not be providing funding for electronic communication systems for the severely communicatively handicapped because they are not interpreting their regulations concerning the funding of prostheses to include such systems. Some speech-language pathologists have played an advocacy role by convincing such administrators that electronic communication systems are prostheses (i.e., communication prostheses) and are thus fundable under existing regulations.

A speech-language pathologist or audiologist can play an advocacy role by providing information to clients or their families that might assist them in obtaining services (or funding) they have been refused, despite their being entitled to them by law. The assumption being made here is that the administrators of a program realize that a person is entitled to services they are refusing to provide, perhaps because their budget is inadequate to cover all of the services they are supposed to fund. A clinician may be able to *discreetly* give the client or family information that could result in the agency's providing the needed services. The word *discreetly* is emphasized because an indiscreet clinician could place himself or herself in a position where the employer would be aware that he or she was functioning as an advocate for the client rather than the employer. Obviously, this would not enhance a clinician's job security.

What advice might a clinician give that could assist a client in obtaining services to which the client is entitled but that he has been refused? Perhaps the most effective strategy would be for the client to *threaten legal action* if the services or funds are not provided. Most government agencies will go to great lengths to avoid such litigation, particularly if they know that they will probably lose. It can be very costly to an agency to lose such litigation because if a court decided that they have to provide services they are not currently providing, it would establish a *precedent* that would be likely to result in requests from others for the services. Hence, the administrators of the agency may view it as potentially less costly to quietly provide the services rather than to risk litigation.

REFERENCES

SCHRIFTGIESSER, K., *The Lobbyists.* Boston: Little, Brown (1951).
The Washington connection: *Asha* interviews Morgan Downey. *Asha,* 23, 480-483 (1981).
The Washington Lobby. Washington, D.C.: Congressional Quarterly (1971).

Appendix A

Representative Release Forms

PERMISSION FOR RELEASE OF INFORMATION

I hereby give my permission for (insert name of institution) to provide information on

_____ to the following:

_____   _____
_____   _____
_____   _____
_____

This information will consist of the following:

_____
_____
_____
_____

Date _____

Signature _____

Check one: _____ Self

_____ Parent

_____ Guardian

Form A-1

PERMISSION FOR REQUEST OF INFORMATION

I hereby give permission to the following:

_____

_____

_____

_____

to release information on _____

to (insert name of institution).

                                      Date _____

                                Signature _____

Check one: _____ Self

              _____ Parent

              _____ Guardian

Form A-2

PERMISSION FOR VIDEOTAPING AND RECORDING CLINICAL WORK

RE: _____

TO: (insert name of institution)

Whereas (insert name of institution), in its speech and hearing habilitation center, wishes to videotape and record therapy sessions and the clinical work conducted at the center for use by (insert name of institution), its students, agents, and employees, therefore, the undersigned hereby grant permission to (insert name of institution) to record on film, tape, or otherwise the first name, likeness, and performance of _____ at the habilitation center for the use of (insert name of institution). This permission will remain in force and effect until revoked in writing by the undersigned.

Date _____

Signature _____

Check one: _____ Self

_____ Parent

_____ Guardian

Form A-3

PERMISSION FOR PUBLICATION OF PHOTOGRAPHS

IN PROMOTIONAL LITERATURE (I.E., MODEL RELEASE)

I hereby give (insert name of institution) the absolute right and permission to copyright and/or publish the photographic portraits or pictures of _____ that were taken on _____, 198_. I agree that the photographs become the exclusive property of (insert name of institution) and I waive all rights thereto.

I waive all rights to inspect and/or approve copy that may be used in conjunction with the photographs and the use to which it may be applied.

The photographs -- whole, in part, or composite -- may be used as (insert name of institution) sees fit in the publication of educational and promotional materials and for any other lawful purpose.

Date _____

Signature _____

Check one: _____ Self

_____ Parent

_____ Guardian

Form A-4

PERMISSION FOR PARTICIPATING IN NONTHERAPEUTIC RESEARCH

TITLE OF PROJECT:

I, _____, hereby consent to participate in the experimental project being conducted by (insert name of institution) where (insert description of task). I have been told that (insert statement of what subject has been told about potential risks). I understand that I may choose to discontinue participation in the project at any time if I so desire. I understand that participation in this project will not necessarily benefit me directly, but that information gained from the project may someday benefit others.

Date _____

Signature _____

Check one: _____ Self

_____ Parent

_____ Guardian

Form A-5

Appendix B

Representative Regulations Governing the Use of Human Subjects

NUREMBERG CODE (1946)*

Note: The Nuremberg Code, which was one of the first attempts to regulate human experimentation, consists of ten points that delimit permissible experimentation on human subjects. It was motivated by abuses in such experimentation that occurred in Nazi Germany during World War II.

1. The voluntary consent of the human subject is absolutely essential. This means that the person involved should have legal capacity to give consent; should be so situated as to be able to exercise free power of choice, without the intervention of any element of force, fraud, deceit, duress, over-reaching, or other ulterior form of constraint or coercion, and should have sufficient knowledge and comprehension of the elements of the subject matter involved as to enable him to make an understanding and enlightened decision. This latter element requires that before the acceptance of an affirmative decision by the experimental subject there should be made known to him the nature, duration, and purpose of the experiment; the method and means by which it is to be conducted, all inconveniences and hazards reasonably to be expected; and the effects upon his health or person which may possibly come from his participation in the experiment.

*Reprinted from "Permissible medical experiments" in *Trials of War Criminals before the Nuremberg Military Tribunals under Control Council Law No. 10: Nuremberg 1946 to April 1949*. Washington, D.C.: U.S. Government Printing Office (no date).

The duty and responsibility for ascertaining the quality of the consent rests upon each individual who initiates, directs or engages in the experiment. It is a personal duty and responsibility which may not be delegated to another with impunity.
2. The experiment should be such as to yield fruitful results for the good of society, unprocurable by other methods or means of study, and not random and unnecessary in nature.
3. The experiment should be so designed and based on the results of animal experimentation and a knowledge of the natural history of the disease or other problem under study that the anticipated results will justify the performance of the experiment.
4. The experiment should be so conducted as to avoid all unnecessary physical and mental suffering and injury.
5. No experiment should be conducted where there is an *a priori* reason to believe that death or disabling injury will occur; except, perhaps, in those experiments where the experimental physicians also serve as subjects.
6. The degree of risk to be taken should never exceed that determined by the humanitarian importance of the problem to be solved by the experiment.
7. Proper preparations should be made and adequate facilities provided to protect the experimental subject against even remote possibilities of injury, disability, or death.
8. The experiment should be conducted only by scientifically qualified persons. The highest degree of skill and care should be required through all stages of the experiment of those who conduct or engage in the experiment.
9. During the course of the experiment the human subject should be at liberty to bring the experiment to an end if he has reached the physical or mental state where continuation of the experiment seems to him to be impossible.
10. During the course of the experiment the scientist in charge must be prepared to terminate the experiment at any stage, if he has probable cause to believe, in the exercise of the good faith, superior skill and careful judgment required of him that a continuation of the experiment is likely to result in injury, disability, or death of the experimental subject.

DECLARATION OF HELSINKI (1964)*

Note: This document has replaced the Nuremberg Code to some extent. The recommendations contained in it for conducting experiments using human subjects have been adopted by the World Medical Association. It represents one of the first attempts by the international scientific community to regulate human experimentation. Though its emphasis is medical, most of the recommendations are applicable to research in speech-language pathology and audiology. You may wish to substitute the word "clinician" for "doctor" while reading it. A somewhat expanded version of this code was adopted by the World Medical Association in 1975.

*Reprinted with permission of *The World Medical Journal.*

Introduction

It is the mission of the doctor to safeguard the health of the people. His knowledge and conscience are dedicated to the fulfillment of this mission. . . .

Because it is essential that the results of laboratory experiments be applied to human beings to further scientific knowledge and to help suffering humanity, the World Medical Association has prepared the following recommendations as a guide to each doctor in clinical research. It must be stressed that the standards as drafted are only a guide to physicians all over the world. Doctors are not relieved from criminal, civil and ethical responsibilities under the laws of their own countries.

In the field of clinical research a fundamental distinction must be recognized between clinical research in which the aim is essentially therapeutic for a patient, and the clinical research, the essential object of which is purely scientific and without therapeutic value to the person subjected to the research.

I. Basic Principles

1. Clinical research must conform to the moral and scientific principles that justify medical research and should be based on laboratory and animal experiments or other scientifically established facts.
2. Clinical research should be conducted only by scientifically qualified persons and under the supervision of a qualified medical man.
3. Clinical research cannot legitimately be carried out unless the importance of the objective is in proportion to the inherent risk to the subject.
4. Every clinical research project should be preceded by careful assessment of inherent risks in comparison to foreseeable benefits to the subject or to others.
5. Special caution should be exercised by the doctor in performing clinical research in which the personality of the subject is liable to be altered by drugs or experimental procedure.

II. Clinical Research Combined with Professional Care

1. In the treatment of the sick person, the doctor must be free to use a new therapeutic measure, if in his judgment it offers hope of saving life, reestablishing health, or alleviating suffering.

    If at all possible, consistent with patient psychology, the doctor should obtain the patient's freely given consent after the patient has been given a full explanation. In case of legal incapacity, consent should also be procured from the legal guardian; in the case of physical incapacity the permission of the legal guardian replaces that of the patient.
2. The doctor can combine clinical research with professional care, the objective being the acquisition of new medical knowledge, only to the extent that clinical research is justified by its therapeutic value for the patient.

III. Non-Therapeutic Clinical Research

1. In the purely scientific application of clinical research carried out on a human being, it is the duty of the doctor to remain the protector of the life and health of that person on whom clinical research is being carried out.
2. The nature, the purpose and the risk of clinical research must be explained to the subject by the doctor.

3a. Clinical research on a human being cannot be undertaken without his free consent after he has been informed; if he is legally incompetent, the consent of the legal guardian should be procured.

3b. The subject of clinical research should be in such a mental, physical and legal state as to be able to exercise fully his power of choice.

3c. Consent should, as a rule, be obtained in writing. However, the responsibility for clinical research always remains with the research worker; it never falls on the subject even after consent is obtained.

4a. The investigator must respect the right of each individual to safeguard his personal integrity, especially if the subject is in a dependent relationship to the investigator.

4b. At any time during the course of clinical research the subject or his guardian should be free to withdraw permission for research to be continued.

The investigator or the investigating team should discontinue the research if in his or their judgment, it may, if continued, be harmful to the individual.

Appendix C

Selected Legislation Relevant to Speech-Language Pathologists and Audiologists

Communication Act of 1934 (47 USCA 151) This act established the Federal Communications Commission, which has been concerned with the telecommunication needs of the deaf (including TTY service).

Consumer Product Warranties (15 USCA 2301, Commerce & Trade) This act established rules governing the contents of warranties. It is relevant to speech-language pathologists and audiologists in their role as dispensers of products such as hearing aids and electronic augmentative communication systems.

Education for All Handicapped Children Act (P.L. 94-142) This act was intended to assure that all handicapped children would have available to them a free appropriate public education, including special education and related services. It has had a profound impact on the programming and delivery of speech, language, and hearing services in the public schools.

Federal Food, Drug, and Cosmetic Act (21 USCA 301) This act was intended to protect consumers from abuse and harm caused by the introduction, adulteration, or misbranding of any food, drug, *device*, or cosmetic in interstate commerce. Hearing aids are classified as a device under this act.

Federal Trade Commission; Promotion of Export Trade and Prevention of Unfair Methods of Competition (15 USCA 41, Commerce & Trade) This act created the Federal Trade Commission, which has attempted to alleviate anticompetitive practices in the hearing aid industry.

Hospital, Nursing Home, Domiciliary, and Medical Care (38 USCA 601, Veterans' Benefits) This act was intended to define eligibility for veterans to receive health-related services in Veterans' Administration and private facilities. The services covered by the act include those provided by speech-language pathologists and audiologists.

Medical Devices Amendment (21 USCA 321) This act was intended to regulate the safety and efficacy of medical devices, including diagnostic and rehabilitative audiometric instrumentation.

Occupational Safety and Health Amendments of 1970 (P.L. 91-596) This act was intended to assure that all working men and women would have a "safe and healthful" work environment, one aspect of which would be an acceptable environmental noise level.

Rehabilitation Act of 1973 (P.L. 93-112) This act was intended to eliminate discriminatory practices against handicapped persons. Section 504 states that "No otherwise qualified handicapped individual in the United States... shall, solely by reason of his handicap, be excluded from participation in, be denied the benefit of, or be subjected to discrimination under any program or activity receiving Federal financial assistance."

Social Security Act (42 USCA 301) This act funds several programs, including Medicare, that will pay for some speech, language, and hearing services for several subgroups of the communicatively handicapped population. These subgroups include crippled children and aged persons (who are eligible for Medicare).

Sherman Antitrust Act (15 USCA 1, Commerce & Trade) This act was intended to prevent corporations and associations from engaging in restraint of trade. It has influenced ASHA's ethical guidelines for dispensing products (e.g., hearing aids) to persons with communicative disorders (see *Asha,* June 1978).

Appendix D

Constitution of the United States

We the People of the United States, in Order to form a more perfect Union, establish Justice, insure domestic Tranquility, provide for the common defence, promote the general Welfare, and secure the Blessings of Liberty to ourselves and our Posterity, do ordain and establish this Constitution for the United States of America.

Article I

Section 1. All legislative Powers herein granted shall be vested in a Congress of the United States, which shall consist of a Senate and House of Representatives.

Section 2. The House of Representatives shall be composed of Members chosen every second Year by the People of the several States, and the Electors in each State shall have the Qualifications requisite for Electors of the most numerous Branch of the State Legislature.

No Person shall be a Representative who shall not have attained to the Age of twenty five Years, and been seven Years a Citizen of the United States, and who shall not, when elected, be an Inhabitant of the State in which he shall be chosen.

Representatives and direct Taxes shall be apportioned among the several States which may be included within this Union, according to their respective Numbers, which shall be determined by adding to the whole Number of free Persons, including those bound to Service for a Term of Years, and excluding Indians not taxed, three fifths of all other Persons. The actual Enumeration shall be made within three Years after the first Meeting of the Congress of the United States, and within every subsequent Term of ten Years, in such Manner as they shall by Law

Reproduced from the 1977/1978 United States Government Manual. Washington, D.C.: U.S. Government Printing Office.

direct. The Number of Representatives shall not exceed one for every thirty Thousand, but each State shall have at Least one Representative; and until such enumeration shall be made, the State of New Hampshire shall be entitled to chuse three, Massachusetts eight, Rhode-Island and Providence Plantations one, Connecticut five, New-York six, New Jersey four, Pennsylvania eight, Delaware one, Maryland six, Virginia ten, North Carolina five, South Carolina five, and Georgia three.

When vacancies happen in the Representation from any State, the Executive Authority thereof shall issue Writs of Election to fill such Vacancies.

The House of Representatives shall chuse their speaker and other Officers; and shall have the sole Power of Impeachment.

Section 3. The Senate of the United States shall be composed of two Senators from each State, chosen by the Legislature thereof, for six Years; and each Senator shall have one Vote.

Immediately after they shall be assembled in Consequence of the first Election, they shall be divided as equally as may be into three Classes. The Seats of the Senators of the first Class shall be vacated at the Expiration of the second Year, of the second Class at the Expiration of the fourth Year, and of the third Class at the Expiration of the sixth Year, so that one third may be chosen every second Year; and if Vacancies happen by Resignation, or otherwise, during the Recess of the Legislature of any State, the Executive thereof may make temporary Appointments until the next Meeting of the Legislature, which shall then fill such Vacancies.

No Person shall be a senator who shall not have attained to the Age of thirty Years, and been nine Years a Citizen of the United States, and who shall not, when elected, be an Inhabitant of that State for which he shall be chosen.

The Vice President of the United States shall be President of the Senate, but shall have no Vote, unless they be equally divided.

The Senate shall chuse their other Officers, and also a President pro tempore, in the Absence of the Vice President, or when he shall exercise the Office of President of the United States.

The Senate shall have the sole Power to try all Impeachments. When sitting for that Purpose, they shall be on Oath or Affirmation. When the President of the United States is tried, the Chief Justice shall preside: And no Person shall be convicted without the Concurrence of two thirds of the Members present.

Judgment in Cases of Impeachment shall not extend further than to removal from Office, and disqualification to hold and enjoy any Office of honor, Trust or Profit under the United States: but the Party convicted shall nevertheless be liable and subject to Indictment, Trial, Judgment and Punishment, according to law.

Section 4. The Times, Places and Manner of holding Elections for Senators and Representatives, shall be prescribed in each State by the Legislature thereof; but the Congress may at any time by Law make or alter such Regulations, except as to the Places of chusing Senators.

The Congress shall assemble at least once in every Year, and such Meeting shall be on the first Monday in December, unless they shall by Law appoint a different Day.

Section 5. Each House shall be the Judge of the Elections, Returns and Qualifications of its own Members, and a Majority of each shall constitute a Quorum to do Business; but a smaller Number may adjourn from day to day, and may be authorized to compel the Attendance of absent Members, in such Manner, and under such Penalties as each House may provide.

Each House may determine the Rules of its Proceedings, punish its Members for disorderly Behaviour, and, with the Concurrence of two thirds, expel a Member.

Each House shall keep a Journal of its Proceedings, and from time to time publish the same, excepting such Parts as may in their Judgment require Secrecy; and the Yeas and Nays of the Members of either House on any question shall, at the Desire of one fifth of those Present, be entered on the Journal.

Neither House, during the Session of Congress, shall, without the Consent of the other, adjourn for more than three days, nor to any other place than that in which the two Houses shall be sitting.

Section 6. The Senators and Representatives shall receive a Compensation for their Services, to be ascertained by Law, and paid out of the Treasury of the United States. They shall in all Cases, except Treason, Felony and Breach of the Peace, be privileged from Arrest during their Attendance at the Session of their respective Houses, and in going to and returning from the same; and for any Speech or Debate in either House, they shall not be questioned in any other Place.

No Senator or Representative shall, during the Time for which he was elected, be appointed to any civil Office under the Authority of the United States, which shall have been created, or the Emoluments whereof shall have been encreased during such time; and no Person holding any Office under the United States, shall be a Member of either House during his Continuance in Office.

Section 7. All Bills for raising Revenue shall originate in the House of Representatives; but the Senate may propose or concur with Amendments as on other Bills.

Every Bill which shall have passed the House of Representatives and the Senate, shall, before it become a Law, be presented to the President of the United States; If he approve he shall sign it, but if not he shall return it, with his Objections to that House in which it shall have originated, who shall enter the Objections at large on their Journal, and proceed to reconsider it. If after such Reconsideration two thirds of that House shall agree to pass the Bill, it shall be sent, together with the Objections, to the other House, by which it shall likewise be reconsidered, and if approved by two thirds of that House, it shall become a Law. But in all such Cases the Votes of both Houses shall be determined by yeas and Nays, and the Names of the Persons voting for and against the Bill shall be entered on the Journal of each House respectively. If any Bill shall not be returned by the President within ten Days (Sundays excepted) after it shall have been presented to him, the Same shall be a Law, in like Manner as if he had signed it, unless the Congress by their Adjournment prevent its Return, in which Case it shall not be a Law.

Every Order, Resolution, or Vote to which the Concurrence of the Senate and House of Representatives may be necessary (except on a question of Adjournment) shall be presented to the President of the United States; and before the Same shall take Effect, shall be approved by him, or being disapproved by him, shall be repassed by two thirds of the Senate and the House of Representatives, according to the Rules and Limitations prescribed in the Case of a Bill.

Section 8. The Congress shall have Power To lay and collect Taxes, Duties, Imposts and Excises, to pay the Debts and provide for the common Defence and general Welfare of the United States; but all Duties, Imposts and Excises shall be uniform throughout the United States;

To borrow Money on the Credit of the United States;

To regulate Commerce with foreign Nations, and among the several States, and with the Indian Tribes;

To establish an uniform Rule of Naturalization, and uniform Laws on the subject of Bankruptcies throughout the United States;

To coin Money, regulate the Value thereof, and of foreign Coin, and fix the Standard of Weights and Measures;

To provide for the Punishment of counterfeiting the Securities and current Coin of the United States;

To establish Post Offices and post Roads;

To promote the Progress of Science and useful Arts, by securing for limited Times to Authors and Inventors the exclusive Right to their respective Writings and Discoveries;

To constitute Tribunals inferior to the supreme Court;

To define and punish Piracies and Felonies committed on the high Seas, and Offences against the Law of Nations;

To declare War, grant Letters of Marque and Reprisal, and make Rules concerning Captures on Land and Water;

To raise and support Armies, but no Appropriation of Money to that Use shall be for a longer Term than two Years;

To provide and maintain a Navy;

To make Rules for the Government and Regulation of the land and naval Forces;

To provide for calling forth the Militia to execute the Laws of the Union, suppress Insurrections and repel Invasions;

To provide for organizing, arming, and disciplining, the Militia, and for governing such Part of them as may be employed in the Service of the United States, reserving to the State respectively, the Appointment of the Officers, and the Authority of training the Militia according to the discipline prescribed by Congress;

To exercise exclusive Legislation in all Cases whatsoever, over such District (not exceeding ten Miles square), as may, by Cession of particular States, and the Acceptance of Congress, become the Seat of the Government of the United States, and to exercise like Authority over all Places purchased by the Consent of the Legislature of the State in which the Same shall be for the Erection of Forts, Magazines, Arsenals, dock-Yards, and other needful Buildings;—And

To make all Laws which shall be necessary and proper for carrying into Execution the foregoing Powers, and all other Powers vested by this Constitution in the Government of the United States, or in any Department or Officer thereof.

Section 9. The Migration or Importation of such Persons as any of the States now existing shall think proper to admit, shall not be prohibited by the Congress prior to the Year one thousand eight hundred and eight, but a Tax or duty may be imposed on such Importation, not exceeding ten dollars for each Person.

The Privilege of the Writ of Habeas Corpus shall not be suspended, unless when in Cases of Rebellion or Invasion the public Safety may require it.

No Bill of Attainder or ex post facto Law shall be passed.

No Capitation, or other direct, Tax shall be laid, unless in Proportion to the Census or Enumeration herein before directed to be taken.

No Tax or Duty shall be laid on Articles exported from any State.

No Preference shall be given by any Regulation of Commerce or Revenue to the Ports of one State over those of another: nor shall Vessels bound to, or from, one State, be obliged to enter, clear, or pay Duties in another.

No Money shall be drawn from the Treasury, but in Consequence of Appropriations made by Law; and a regular Statement and Account of the Receipts and Expenditures of all public Money shall be published from time to time.

No Title of Nobility shall be granted by the United States: And no Person holding any Office of Profit or Trust under them, shall, without the Consent of the Congress, accept of any present, Emolument, Office, or Title, of any kind whatever, from any King, Prince, or foreign State.

Section 10. No State shall enter into any Treaty, Alliance, or Confederation; grant Letters of Marque and Reprisal; coin Money; emit Bills of Credit; make any Thing but gold and silver Coin a Tender in Payment of Debts; pass any Bill of Attainder, ex post facto Law, or Law impairing the Obligation of Contracts, or grant any Title of Nobility.

No State shall, without the Consent of the Congress, lay any Imposts or Duties on Imports or Exports, except what may be absolutely necessary for executing it's inspection Laws: and the net Produce of all Duties and Imposts, laid by any State on Imports or Exports, shall be for the Use of the Treasury of the United States; and all such Laws shall be subject to the Revision and Controul of the Congress.

No State shall, without the Consent of Congress, lay any Duty of Tonnage, keep Troops, or Ships of War in time of Peace, enter into any Agreement or Compact with another State, or with a foreign Power, or engage in War, unless actually invaded, or in such imminent Danger as will not admit of delay.

Article II

Section 1. The executive Power shall be vested in a President of the United States of America. He shall hold his Office during the Term of four Years, and, together with the Vice President, chosen for the same term, be elected, as follows

Each State shall appoint, in such Manner as the Legislature thereof may direct, a Number of Electors, equal to the whole Number of Senators and Representatives to which the State may be entitled in the Congress: but no Senator or Representative, or Person holding an Office of Trust or Profit under the United States, shall be appointed an Elector.

The Electors shall meet in their respective States, and vote by Ballot for two Persons, of whom one at least shall not be an Inhabitant of the same State with themselves. And they shall make a List of all the Persons voted for, and of the Number of Votes for each; which List they shall sign and certify, and transmit sealed to the Seat of the Government of the United States, directed to the President of the Senate. The President of the Senate shall, in the Presence of the Senate and House of Representatives, open all the Certificates, and the Votes shall then be counted. The Person having the greatest Number of Votes shall be the President, if such Number be a Majority of the whole Number of Electors appointed; and if there be more than one who have such Majority, and have an equal Number of Votes, then the House of Representatives shall immediately chuse by Ballot one of them for President: and if no Person have a Majority, then from the five highest on the List the said House shall in like Manner chuse the President. But in chusing the President, the Votes shall be taken by States, the Representation from each State having one Vote; A quorum for this Purpose shall consist of a Member or Members from two thirds of the States, and a Majority of all the States shall be necessary to a Choice. In every Case, after the Choice of the President, the Person having the greatest Number of Votes of the Electors shall be the Vice President. But if there should remain two or more who have equal Votes, the Senate shall chuse from them by Ballot the Vice President.

The Congress may determine the Time of chusing the Electors, and the Day on which they shall give their Votes; which Day shall be the same throughout the United States.

No Person except a natural born Citizen, or a Citizen of the United States, at the time of the Adoption of this Constitution, shall be eligible to the Office of President; neither shall any Person be eligible to that Office who shall not have attained to the Age of thirty five Years, and been fourteen Years a Resident within the United States.

In Case of the Removal of the President from Office, or of his Death, Resignation, or Inability to discharge the Powers and Duties of the said Office, the Same shall devolve on the Vice President, and the Congress may by Law provide for the Case of Removal, Death, Resignation or Inability, both of the President and Vice President, declaring what Officer shall then act as President, and such Officer shall act accordingly, until the Disability be removed, or a President shall be elected.

The President shall, at stated Times, receive for his Services, a Compensation, which shall neither be encreased nor diminished during the Period for which he shall have been elected, and he shall not receive within that Period any other Emolument from the United States, or any of them.

Before he enter on the Execution of his Office, he shall take the following Oath or Affirmation:—"I do solemnly swear (or affirm) that I will faithfully execute the Office of President of the United States, and will to the best of my Ability, preserve, protect and defend the Constitution of the United States."

Section 2. The President shall be Commander in Chief of the Army and Navy of the United States, and of the Militia of the several States, when called into the actual Service of the United States; he may require the Opinion, in writing, of the principal Officer in each of the executive Departments, upon any Subject relating to the Duties of their respective Offices, and he shall have Power to grant Reprieves and Pardons for Offences against the United States, except in Cases of Impeachment.

He shall have Power, by and with the Advice and Consent of the Senate, to make Treaties, provided two thirds of the Senators present concur; and he shall nominate, and by and with the Advice and Consent of the Senate, shall appoint Ambassadors, other public Ministers and Consuls, Judges of the supreme Court, and all other Officers of the United States, whose Appointments are not herein otherwise provided for, and which shall be established by Law: but the Congress may by Law vest the Appointment of such inferior Officers, as they think proper, in the President alone, in the Courts of Law, or in the Heads of Departments.

The President shall have Power to fill up all Vacancies that may happen during the Recess of the Senate, by granting Commissions which shall expire at the End of their next Session.

Section 3. He shall from time to time give to the Congress Information of the State of the Union, and recommend to their Consideration such Measures as he shall judge necessary and expedient; he may, on extraordinary Occasions, convene both Houses, or either of them, and in Case of Disagreement between them, with Respect to the Time of Adjournment, he may adjourn them to such Time as he shall think proper; he shall receive Ambassadors and other public Ministers; he shall take Care that the Laws be faithfully executed, and shall Commission all the Officers of the United States.

Section 4. The President, Vice President and all civil Officers of the United States, shall be removed from Office on Impeachment for, and Conviction of, Treason, Bribery, or other High Crimes and Misdemeanors.

Article III

Section 1. The judicial Power of the United States, shall be vested in one supreme Court, and in such inferior Courts as the Congress may from time to time ordain and establish. The Judges, both of the supreme and inferior Courts, shall hold their

Offices during good Behavior, and shall, at stated Times, receive for their Services, a Compensation, which shall not be diminished during their Continuance in Office.

Section 2. The judicial Power shall extend to all Cases, in Law and Equity, arising under this Constitution, the Laws of the United States, and Treaties made, or which shall be made, under their Authority;—to all Cases affecting Ambassadors, other public Ministers and Consuls;—to all Cases of admiralty and maritime Jurisdiction;—to Controversies to which the United States shall be a Party;—to Controversies between two or more States; between a State and Citizens of another State;—between Citizens of different States;—between Citizens of the same State claiming Lands under Grants of different States, and between a State, or the Citizens thereof, and foreign States, Citizens or Subjects.

In all Cases affecting Ambassadors, other public Ministers and Consuls, and those in which a State shall be Party, the supreme Court shall have original Jurisdiction. In all the other Cases before mentioned, the supreme Court shall have appellate Jurisdiction, both as to Law and Fact, with such Exceptions, and under such Regulations as the Congress shall make.

The Trial of all Crimes, except in Cases of Impeachment, shall be by Jury; and such Trial shall be held in the State where the said Crimes shall have been committed; but when not committed within any State, the Trial shall be at such Place or Places as the Congress may by Law have directed.

Section 3. Treason against the United States, shall consist only in levying War against them, or in adhering to their Enemies, giving them Aid and Comfort. No Person shall be convicted of Treason unless on the Testimony of two Witnesses to the same overt Act, or on Confession in open Court.

The Congress shall have Power to declare the Punishment of Treason, but no Attainder of Treason shall work Corruption of Blood, or Forefeiture except during the Life of the Person attainted.

Article IV

Section 1. Full Faith and Credit shall be given in each State to the public Acts, Records, and judicial Proceedings of every other State. And the Congress may by general Laws prescribe the Manner in which such Acts, Records and Proceedings shall be proved, and the Effect thereof.

Section 2. The Citizens of each State shall be entitled to all Privileges and Immunities of Citizens in the several States.

A person charged in any State with Treason, Felony, or other Crime, who shall flee from Justice, and be found in another State, shall on Demand of the executive Authority of the State from which he fled, be delivered up, to be removed to the State having Jurisdiction of the Crime.

No person held to Service or Labour in one State, under the Laws thereof, escaping into another, shall, in Consequence of any Law or Regulation therein, be discharged from such Service or Labour, but shall be delivered up on Claim of the Party to whom such Service or Labour may be due.

Section 3. New States may be admitted by the Congress into this Union; but no new State shall be formed or erected within the Jurisdiction of any other State; nor any State be formed by the Junction of two or more States, or Parts of States, without the Consent of the Legislatures of the States concerned as well as of the Congress.

The Congress shall have Power to dispose of and make all needful Rules and Regulations respecting the Territory or other Property belonging to the United States;

and nothing in this Constitution shall be so construed as to Prejudice any Claims of the United States, or of any particular State.

Section 4. The United States shall guarantee to every State in this Union a Republican Form of Government, and shall protect each of them against Invasion; and on Application of the Legislature, or of the Executive (when the Legislature cannot be convened) against domestic Violence.

Article V

The Congress, whenever two thirds of both Houses shall deem it necessary, shall propose Amendments to this Constitution, or, on the Application of the Legislatures of two thirds of the several States, shall call a Convention for proposing Amendments, which, in either Case, shall be valid to all Intents and Purposes, as Part of this Constitution, when ratified by the Legislatures of three fourths of the several States, or by Conventions in three fourths thereof, as the one or the other Mode of Ratification may be proposed by the Congress; Provided that no Amendment which may be made prior to the Year One thousand eight hundred and eight shall in any Manner affect the first and fourth Clauses in the Ninth Section of the first Article; and that no State, without its Consent, shall be deprived of its equal Suffrage in the Senate.

Article VI

All Debts contracted and Engagements entered into, before the Adoption of this Constitution, shall be as valid against the United States under this Constitution, as under the Confederation.

This Constitution, and the Laws of the United States which shall be made in Pursuance thereof; and all Treaties made, or which shall be made, under the Authority of the United States, shall be the supreme Law of the Land; and the Judges in every State shall be bound thereby, any Thing in the Constitution or Laws of any State to the Contrary notwithstanding.

The Senators and Representatives before mentioned, and the Members of the several State Legislatures, and all executive and judicial Officers, both of the United States and of the several States, shall be bound by Oath or Affirmation, to support this Constitution; but no religious Test shall ever be required as a Qualification to any Office or public Trust under the United States.

Article VII

The Ratification of the Conventions of nine States, shall be sufficient for the Establishment of this Constitution between the States so ratifying the Same.

> DONE in Convention by the Unanimous Consent of the States present the Seventeenth Day of September in the Year of our Lord one thousand seven hundred and Eighty seven and of the Independence of the United States of America the Twelfth IN WITNESS WHEREOF We have hereunto subscribed our Names,
>
> Ge. WASHINGTON–Presidt.
and deputy from Virginia

New Hampshire	John Langdon Nicholas Gilman
Massachusetts	Nathaniel Gorham Rufus King
Connecticut	W Sam Johnson Roger Sherman
New York	Alexander Hamilton
New Jersey	Wil: Livingston David Brearley. Wm. Paterson. Jona: Dayton
Pennsylvania	B Franklin Thomas Mifflin Robt Morris Geo. Clymer Thos FitzSimons Jared Ingersoll James Wilson Gouv Morris
Delaware	Geo: Read Gunning Bedford jun John Dickinson Richard Bassett Jaco: Broom
Maryland	James McHenry Dan of St Thos Jenifer Danl Carroll
Virginia	John Blair— James Madison Jr.
North Carolina	Wm Blount Richd Dobbs Spaight. Hu Williamson
South Carolina	J. Rutledge Charles Cotesworth Pinckney Charles Pinckney Pierce Butler.
Georgia	William Few Abr Baldwin

Amendments

(The first 10 Amendments were ratified December 15, 1791, and form what is known as the "Bill of Rights")

Amendment 1

Congress shall make no law respecting an establishment of religion, or prohibiting the free exercise thereof; or abridging the freedom of speech, or of the press; or the right of the people peaceably to assemble, and to petition the Government for a redress of grievances.

Amendment 2

A well regulated Militia, being necessary to the security of a free State, the right of the people to keep and bear Arms, shall not be infringed.

Amendment 3

No Soldier shall, in time of peace be quartered in any house, without the consent of the Owner, nor in time of war, but in a manner to be prescribed by law.

Amendment 4

The right of the people to be secure in their persons, houses, papers, and effects, against unreasonable searches and seizures, shall not be violated, and no Warrants shall issue, but upon probable cause, supported by Oath or affirmation, and particularly describing the place to be searched, and the persons or things to be seized.

Amendment 5

No person shall be held to answer for a capital, or otherwise infamous crime, unless on a presentment or indictment of a Grand Jury, except in cases arising in the land or naval forces, or in the Militia, when in actual service in time of War or public danger; nor shall any person be subject for the same offence to be twice put in jeopardy of life or limb; nor shall be compelled in any criminal case to be a witness against himself, nor be deprived of life, liberty, or property, without due process of law; nor shall private property be taken for public use, without just compensation.

Amendment 6

In all criminal prosecutions, the accused shall enjoy the right to a speedy and public trial, by an impartial jury of the State and district wherein the crime shall have been committed, which district shall have been previously ascertained by law, and to be informed of the nature and cause of the accusation; to be confronted with the witnesses against him; to have compulsory process for obtaining witnesses in his favor, and to have the Assistance of Counsel for his defence.

Amendment 7

In Suits at common law, where the value in controversy shall exceed twenty dollars, the right of trial by jury shall be preserved, and no fact tried by a jury, shall be otherwise re-examined in any Court of the United States, than according to the rules of the common law.

Amendment 8

Excessive bail shall not be required, nor excessive fines imposed, nor cruel and unusual punishments inflicted.

Amendment 9

The enumeration in the Constitution, of certain rights, shall not be construed to deny or disparage others retained by the people.

Amendment 10

The powers not delegated to the United States by the Constitution, nor prohibited by it to the States, are reserved to the States respectively, or to the people.

Amendment 11

(Ratified February 7, 1795)

The Judicial power of the United States shall not be construed to extend to any suit in law or equity, commenced or prosecuted against one of the United States by Citizens of another State, or by Citizens or Subjects of any Foreign State.

Amendment 12

(Ratified July 27, 1804)

The Electors shall meet in their respective states and vote by ballot for President and Vice-President, one of whom, at least, shall not be an inhabitant of the same state with themselves; they shall name in their ballots the person voted for as President, and in district ballots the person voted for as Vice-President, and they shall make distinct lists of all persons voted for as President, and of all persons voted for as Vice-President, and of the number of votes for each, which lists they shall sign and certify, and transmit sealed to the seat of the government of the United States, directed to the President of the Senate;—The President of the Senate shall, in the presence of the Senate and House of Representatives, open all the certificates and the votes shall then be counted;—The person having the greatest number of votes for President, shall be the President, if such number be a majority of the whole number of Electors appointed; and if no person have such majority, then from the persons having the highest numbers not exceeding three on the list of those voted for as President, the House of Representatives shall choose immediately, by ballot, the President. But in choosing the President, the votes shall be taken by states, the representation from each state having one vote; a quorum for this purpose shall consist of a member or members from two-thirds of the states, and a majority of all the states shall be necessary to a choice. And if the House of Representatives shall not choose a President whenever the right of choice shall devolve upon them, before the fourth day of March next following, then the Vice-President shall act as President, as in the case of the death of other constitutional disability of the President.—The person having the greatest number of votes as Vice-President, shall be the Vice-President, if such number be a majority of the whole number of Electors appointed, and if no person have a majority, then from the two highest numbers on the list, the Senate shall choose the Vice-President; a quorum for the purpose shall consist of two-thirds of the whole number of Senators, and a majority of the whole number shall be necessary to a choice. But no person constitutionally ineligible to the office of President shall be eligible to that of Vice-President of the United States.

Amendment 13

(Ratified December 6, 1865)

Section 1. Neither slavery nor involuntary servitude, except as a punishment for crime whereof the party shall have been duly convicted, shall exist within the United States, or any place subject to their jurisdiction.

Section 2. Congress shall have power to enforce this article by appropriate legislation.

Amendment 14

(Ratified July 9, 1868)

Section 1. All persons born or naturalized in the United States, and subject to the jurisdiction thereof, are citizens of the United States and of the State wherein they reside. No State shall make or enforce any law which shall abridge the privileges or immunities of citizens of the United States; nor shall any State deprive any person of life, liberty, or property, without due process of law; nor deny to any person within its jurisdiction the equal protection of the laws.

Section 2. Representatives shall be apportioned among the several States according to their respective numbers, counting the whole number of persons in each State, excluding Indians not taxed. But when the right to vote at any election for the choice of electors for President and Vice President of the United States, Representatives in Congress, the Executive and Judicial officers of a State, or the members of the Legislature thereof, is denied to any of the male inhabitants of such State, being twenty-one years of age, and citizens of the United States, or in any way abridged, except for participation in rebellion, or other crime, the basis of representation therein shall be reduced in the proportion which the number of such male citizens shall bear to the whole number of male citizens twenty-one years of age in such State.

Section 3. No person shall be a Senator or Representative in Congress, or elector of President and Vice President, or hold any office, civil or military, under the United States, or under any State, who, having previously taken an oath, as a member of Congress, or as an officer of the United States, or as a member of any State legislature, or as an executive or judicial officer of any State, to support the Constitution of the United States, shall have engaged in insurrection or rebellion against the same, or given aid or comfort to the enemies thereof. But Congress may by a vote of two-thirds of each House, remove such disability.

Section 4. The validity of the public debt of the United States, authorized by law, including debts incurred for payment of pensions and bounties for services in suppressing insurrection or rebellion, shall not be questioned. But neither the United States nor any State shall assume or pay any debt or obligation incurred in aid of insurrection or rebellion against the United States, or any claim for the loss or emancipation of any slave; but all such debts, obligations and claims shall be held illegal and void.

Section 5. The Congress shall have power to enforce, by appropriate legislation, the provisions of this article.

Amendment 15

(Ratified February 3, 1870)

Section 1. The right of citizens of the United States to vote shall not be denied or abridged by the United States or by any State on account of race, color, or previous condition of servitude.

Section 2. The Congress shall have power to enforce this article by appropriate legislation.

Amendment 16

(Ratified February 3, 1913)

The Congress shall have power to lay and collect taxes on incomes, from whatever source derived, without apportionment among the several States, and without regard to any census or enumeration.

Amendment 17

(Ratified April 8, 1913)

The Senate of the United States shall be composed of two Senators from each State, elected by the people thereof for six years; and each Senator shall have one vote. The electors in each State shall have the qualifications requisite for electors of the most numerous branch of the State legislatures.

When vacancies happen in the representation of any State in the Senate, the executive authority of such State shall issue writs of election to fill such vacancies; *Provided*, That the legislature of any State may empower the executive thereof to make temporary appointments until the people fill the vacancies by election as the legislature may direct.

This amendment shall not be so construed as to affect the election or term of any Senator chosen before it becomes valid as part of the Constitution.

Amendment 18

(Ratified January 16, 1919. Repealed December 5, 1933 by Amendment 21)

Section 1. After one year from the ratification of this article the manufacture, sale, or transportation of intoxicating liquors within, the importation thereof into, or the exportation thereof from the United States and all territory subject to the jurisdiction thereof for beverage purposes is hereby prohibited.

Section 2. The Congress and the several States shall have concurrent power to enforce this article by appropriate legislation.

Section 3. This article shall be inoperative unless it shall have been ratified as an amendment to the Constitution by the legislatures of the several States as provided in the Constitution, within seven years from the date of the submission hereof to the States by the Congress.

Amendment 19

(Ratified August 18, 1920)

The right of citizens of the United States to vote shall not be denied or abridged by the United States or by any State on account of sex.

Congress shall have power to enforce this article by appropriate legislation.

Amendment 20

(Ratified January 23, 1933)

Section 1. The terms of the President and Vice President shall end at noon on the 20th day of January, and the terms of Senators and Representatives at noon on the 3d day of January, of the years in which such terms would have ended if this article had not been ratified; and the terms of their successors shall then begin.

Section 2. The Congress shall assemble at least once in every year, and such meeting shall begin at noon on the 3d day of January, unless they shall by law appoint a different day.

Section 3. If, at the time fixed for the beginning of the term of the President, the President elect shall have died, the Vice President elect shall become President. If a President shall not have been chosen before the time fixed for the beginning of his term, or if the President elect shall have failed to qualify, then the Vice President elect shall act as President until a President shall have qualified; and the Congress may by law provide for the case wherein neither a President elect nor a Vice President elect shall have qualified, declaring who shall then act as President, or the manner in which one who is to act shall be selected, and such person shall act accordingly until a President or Vice President shall have qualified.

Section 4. The Congress may by law provide for the case of the death of any of the persons from whom the House of Representatives may choose a President whenever the right of choice shall have devolved upon them, and for the case of the death of any of the persons from whom the Senate may choose a Vice President whenever the right of choice shall have devolved upon them.

Section 5. Sections 1 and 2 shall take effect on the 15th day of October following the ratification of this article.

Section 6. This article shall be inoperative unless it shall have been ratified as an amendment to the Constitution by the legislatures of three-fourths of the several States within seven years from the date of its submission.

Amendment 21

(Ratified December 5, 1933)

Section 1. The eighteenth article of amendment to the Constitution of the United States is hereby repealed.

Section 2. The transportation or importation into any State, Territory, or possession of the United States for delivery or use therein of intoxicating liquors, in violation of the laws thereof, is hereby prohibited.

Section 3. This article shall be inoperative unless it shall have been ratified as an amendment to the Constitution by conventions in the several States, as provided in the Constitution, within seven years from the date of the submission hereof to the States by the Congress.

Amendment 22

(Ratified February 27, 1951)

Section 1. No person shall be elected to the office of the President more than twice, and no person who has held the office of President, or acted as President, for more than two years of a term to which some other person was elected President shall be elected to the office of the President more than once. But this Article shall not apply to any person holding the office of President when this Article was proposed by the Congress, and shall not prevent any person who may be holding the office of President, or acting as President, during the term within which this Article becomes operative from holding the office of President or acting as President during the remainder of such term.

Section 2. This article shall be inoperative unless it shall have been ratified as an amendment to the Constitution by the legislatures of three-fourths of the several States within seven years from the date of its submission to the States by the Congress.

Amendment 23

(Ratified March 29, 1961)

Section 1. The District constituting the seat of Government of the United States shall appoint in such manner as the Congress may direct:

A number of electors of President and Vice President equal to the whole number of Senators and Representatives in Congress to which the District would be entitled if it were a State, but in no event more than the least populous State; they shall be in addition to those appointed by the States, but they shall be considered, for the purposes of the election of President and Vice President, to be electors appointed by a State; and they shall meet in the District and perform such duties as provided by the twelfth article of amendment.

Section 2. The Congress shall have power to enforce this article by appropriate legislation.

Amendment 24

(Ratified January 23, 1964)

Section 1. The right of citizens of the United States to vote in any primary or other election for President or Vice President, for electors for President or Vice President, or for Senator or Representative in Congress, shall not be denied or abridged by the United States or any State by reason of failure to pay any poll tax or other tax.

Section 2. The Congress shall have power to enforce this article by appropriate legislation.

Amendment 25

(Ratified February 10, 1967)

Section 1. In case of the removal of the President from office or of his death or resignation, the Vice President shall become President.

Section 2. Whenever there is a vacancy in the office of the Vice President, the President shall nominate a Vice President who shall take office upon confirmation by a majority vote of both Houses of Congress.

Section 3. Whenever the President transmits to the President pro tempore of the Senate and the Speaker of the House of Representatives his written declaration that he is unable to discharge the powers and duties of his office, and until he transmits to them a written declaration to the contrary, such powers and duties shall be discharged by the Vice President as Acting President.

Section 4. Whenever the Vice President and a majority of either the principal officers of the executive departments or of such other body as Congress may by law provide, transmit to the President pro tempore of the Senate and the Speaker of the House of Representatives their written declaration that the President is unable to discharge the powers and duties of his office, the Vice President shall immediately assume the powers and duties of the office as Acting President.

Thereafter, when the President transmits to the President pro tempore of the Senate and the Speaker of the House of Representatives his written declaration that no inability exists, he shall resume the powers and duties of his office unless the Vice President and a majority of either the principal officers of the executive department or of such other body as Congress may by law provide, transmit within four days to the President pro tempore of the Senate and the Speaker of the House of Representatives their written declaration that the President is unable to discharge the powers and duties of his office. Thereupon Congress shall decide the issue, assembling within forty-eight hours for that purpose if not in session. If the Congress, within twenty-one days after receipt of the latter written declaration, or, if Congress is not in session, within twenty-one days after Congress is required to assemble, determines by two-thirds vote of both Houses that the President is unable to discharge the powers and duties of his office, the Vice President shall continue to discharge the same as Acting President; otherwise, the President shall resume the powers and duties of his office.

Amendment 26

(Ratified July 1, 1971)

Section 1. The right of citizens of the United States, who are eighteen years of age or older, to vote shall not be denied or abridged by the United States or by any State on account of age.

Section 2. The Congress shall have the power to enforce this article by appropriate legislation.

Appendix E

Selected Ethical Codes of the American Speech-Language-Hearing Association 1930–1979

PRINCIPLES OF ETHICS* (of the American Society for the Study of Disorders of Speech) (1930)

The Society proposes the following principles of ethics as an advisory instrument for the selection of new members, and for the professional guidance of present members.

Section I—Duties of Members to the Society. Members shall regard it as their duty and privilege to uphold the dignity and honor of the Society, to promote its interests and the welfare of its members, and to extend its sphere of usefulness whenever and wherever possible. They shall strive for the preservation and integrity of the Society through the practice of high personal standards of excellence in the pursuit of speech correction work, and shall seek to inspire in the public generally an impression of their dependability, culture, knowledge of techniques, and breadth of vision.

Section II—Secrecy. The obligation of secrecy so far as revelation of confidences of speech patients is concerned shall be regarded as a duty of members. Secrecy regarding methods and techniques, however, is opposed to the best interests of the Society; therefore each member shall attempt to extend the benefits of

*This statement of ethical principles was quoted from Paden, 1970, pp. 74-75.

new methods, techniques, practical results, and experimental evidence to every member of the Society.

Section III—Unethical Practices. It shall be considered unethical:

1. To guarantee to cure any disorder of speech.
2. To offer in advance to refund any part of a person's tuition if his disorder of speech is not arrested.
3. To make "rash promises," difficult of fulfillment, in order to secure pupils or patients.
4. To employ blatant or untruthful methods of self-advertising.
5. To advertise to correct disorders of speech entirely by correspondence.
6. To seek self-advancement by attacking the work of other members of the Society in such a way as might injure their standing and reputation. Reproaches or criticisms should be sympathetically discussed with the member involved.
7. For persons who do not hold a medical degree to attempt to deal exclusively with speech patients requiring medical treatment without the advice or the authority of a physician.
8. To extend the time of treatment beyond the time when one should recognize his inability to effect further improvement.
9. To charge exorbitant fees for treatment.

CODE OF ETHICS OF THE AMERICAN SPEECH AND HEARING ASSOCIATION (1951)*

Section 1. Ethical Responsibilities of Members and Associates

The American Speech and Hearing Association is composed of persons having varying interests and professional duties, but certain broad ethical principles apply to the entire membership. The application of these principles to individual cases will depend on the particular circumstances of the professional duties and status of the persons involved.

It is convenient to divide the ethical responsibilities of persons in clinical professions into (1) those duties arising out of the relation between the professional worker and the person who seeks his assistance; (2) duties owed to other professional workers; and (3) obligations to society. These classifications are arbitrary, for actually the duties and responsibilities of the professional worker are indivisible. Any one of these ethical duties clearly implies the other two.

A. The most frequent professional relationship involving Members of ASHA is that of therapist to patient. The ethical responsibilities of this relationship demand that the welfare of the patient be considered paramount. Accordingly, the therapist must possess suitable qualifications for engaging in clinical work. Measures of such qualifications are provided by the Association's program for certification of the clinical competence of Members. The therapist must use every resource available,

*Reprinted from *Journal of Speech and Hearing Disorders,* 1952, pp. 255-256.

including referral to other specialists as needed, to effect as great improvement as possible in the shortest time consistent with good professional practice. Every precaution must be taken against causing any sort of injury to the patient. These general principles are understood and accepted by the profession and the public alike. Their application is the daily task of every professional clinical worker.

Another frequent professional relationship of ASHA Members and Associates is that of teacher to student. The broad ethical responsibilities of the teacher who is a Member or Associate of ASHA are in no way different from those of any other teacher, and no special statement of ethical requirements is in order.

B. The duties owed by Members and Associates to other professional workers are many. They should disseminate results of research and developments in speech and hearing therapy. They should avoid personal controversy, but should seek the freest professional discussion of all theoretical and practical issues. They should establish harmonious relationships with members of other professions, and should especially endeavor to inform them concerning the services that can be rendered by speech and hearing therapists. They should strive to promote the status of ASHA, of the professions of speech and hearing therapy, and of all therapy for and research concerning handicapping conditions.

C. The duties owed to society include first all the obligations of good citizenship which devolve upon members of human society. As persons with special training, ASHA Members and Associates have additional special responsibilities. They should help in the education of the public regarding speech and hearing problems and other matters lying within their professional competence. They should seek to provide and expand services to persons with speech and hearing handicaps, and assist in establishing high professional standards for such programs.

Section 2. Unethical practices.

A. It shall be considered unethical:

1. To guarantee the results of any speech or hearing consultative or therapeutic procedure. Any guarantee of any sort, express or implied, oral or written, is contrary to professional ethics. A therapist may always make a reasonable statement of prognosis, but a 'cure' or other specific favorable outcome is dependent upon many factors outside the therapist's control. Hence any warranty is deceptive and unethical.

2. To employ blatant or sensational advertising. The only form of advertising permissible is the so-called 'business card,' consisting of the name of the person or institution, the type of therapy offered, office hours, address, and telephone number. The words 'type of therapy' refer to such phrases as 'Speech Therapy,' 'Speech and Hearing Therapy,' 'Disorders of Speech,' and similar phrases. Members not holding clinical certification are expressly forbidden to use the name of the Association in advertising or any other professional promotion.

3. To diagnose or treat speech or hearing defects by correspondence. This does not preclude correspondence follow-up of patients previously seen personally.

4. To violate the patient's confidence by revealing any information obtained from or about him without his express permission. Case records must not be used in teaching in such a way as to permit identification of their subjects.

5. To write or say anything which may discredit professional colleagues or members of allied professions other than that based on adequate and objective evaluation of their work.

6. To exploit patients (a) by accepting for treatment patients whose defects cannot reasonably be expected to improve under therapy offered; (b) by continuing therapy unnecessarily; (c) by charging exorbitant fees.

7. To deal with speech patients requiring medical treatment without the advice of a physician.

8. For any student in training, whether on the undergraduate or the graduate level, to treat speech or hearing patients except as this treatment is given under competent supervision and as part of the training program. It will not, however, be considered unethical for a graduate student who holds a Basic Certificate to engage in part-time speech or hearing therapy which is not part of the training program, provided that explicit approval of the director of such training program is secured in advance. A person holding a full-time clinical position and taking part-time graduate work is not, for the purpose of this Section, regarded as a student in training.

9. For any unqualified Member or Associate to treat speech or hearing patients, except under the supervision of one who is properly qualified.

10. To accept compensation from a dealer in prosthetic or other devices for recommending any particular device.

B. In addition to those which have been listed, other practices or actions might have an undesirable effect upon the patient, on relations with other professional personnel, or upon society, and would thus be unethical. It shall be the duty of the Committee on Ethical Practice to decide, in the light of all information it can collect, whether any specific act is in violation of the spirit of these Principles of Ethics.

CODE OF ETHICS OF THE AMERICAN SPEECH-LANGUAGE-HEARING ASSOCIATION (REVISED JANUARY 1, 1979)*

Preamble

The preservation of the highest standards of integrity and ethical principles is vital to the successful discharge of the professional responsibilities of all speech-language pathologists and audiologists. This Code of Ethics has been promulgated by the Association in an effort to stress the fundamental rules considered essential to this basic purpose. Any action that is in violation of the spirit and purpose of this Code shall be considered unethical. Failure to specify any particular responsibility or practice in this Code of Ethics should not be construed as denial of the existence of other responsibilities or practices.

The fundamental rules of ethical conduct are described in three categories: Principles of Ethics, Ethical Proscriptions, Matters of Professional Propriety.

1. *Principles of Ethics.* Six Principles serve as a basis for the ethical evaluation of professional conduct and form the underlying moral basis for the Code of Ethics. Individuals[1] subscribing to this Code shall observe these principles as affirmative obligations under all conditions of professional activity.

2. *Ethical Proscriptions.* Ethical Proscriptions are formal statements of prohibitions that are derived from the Principles of Ethics.

3. *Matters of Professional Propriety.* Matters of Professional Propriety

*Reprinted from the *1980 ASHA Membership Directory.*

[1] "Individuals" refers to all Members of the American Speech-Language-Hearing Association and non-members who hold Certificates of Clinical Competence from this Association.

represent guidelines of conduct designed to promote the public interest and thereby better inform the public and particularly the persons in need of speech-language pathology and audiology services as to the availability and the rules regarding the delivery of those services.

Principles of Ethics I

Individuals shall hold paramount the welfare of persons served professionally.

A. Individuals shall use every resource available, including referral to other specialists as needed, to provide the best service possible.

B. Individuals shall fully inform persons served of the nature and possible effects of the services.

C. Individuals shall fully inform subjects participating in research or teaching activities of the nature and possible effects of these activities.

D. Individuals' fees shall be commensurate with services rendered.

E. Individuals shall provide appropriate access to records of persons served professionally.

F. Individuals shall take all reasonable precautions to avoid injuring persons in the delivery of professional services.

G. Individuals shall evaluate services rendered to determine effectiveness.

Ethical Proscriptions 1. Individuals must not exploit persons in the delivery of professional services, including accepting persons for treatment when benefit cannot reasonably be expected or continuing treatment unnecessarily.

2. Individuals must not guarantee the results of any therapeutic procedures directly or by implication. A reasonable statement of prognosis may be made, but caution must be exercised not to mislead persons served professionally to expect results that cannot be predicted from sound evidence.

3. Individuals must not use persons for teaching or research in a manner that constitutes invasion of privacy or fails to afford informed free choice to participate.

4. Individuals must not evaluate or treat speech, language or hearing disorders except in a professional relationship. They must not evaluate or treat solely by correspondence. This does not preclude follow-up correspondence with persons previously seen, nor providing them with general information of an educational nature.

5. Individuals must not reveal to unauthorized persons any professional or personal information obtained from the person served professionally, unless required by law or unless necessary to protect the welfare of the person or the community.

6. Individuals must not discriminate in the delivery of professional services on any basis that is unjustifiable or irrelevant to the need for and potential benefit from such services, such as race, sex or religion.

7. Individuals must not charge for services not rendered.

Principle of Ethics II

Individuals shall maintain high standards of professional competence.

A. Individuals engaging in clinical practice shall possess appropriate qualifications which are provided by the Association's program for certification of clinical competence.

B. Individuals shall continue their professional development throughout their careers.

C. Individuals shall identify competent, dependable referral sources for persons served professionally.

D. Individuals shall maintain adequate records of professional services rendered.

Ethical Proscriptions 1. Individuals must neither provide services nor supervision of services for which they have not been properly prepared, nor permit services to be provided by any of their staff who are not properly prepared.

2. Individuals must not provide clinical services by prescription of anyone who does not hold the Certificate of Clinical Competence.

3. Individuals must not delegate any service requiring the professional competence of a certified clinician to anyone unqualified.

4. Individuals must not offer clinical services by supportive personnel for whom they do not provide appropriate supervision and assume full responsiblity.

5. Individuals must not require anyone under their supervision to engage in any practice that is a violation of the Code of Ethics.

Principle of Ethics III

Individuals' statements to persons served professionally and to the public shall provide accurate information about the nature and management of communicative disorders, and about the profession and services rendered by its practitioners.

Ethical Proscriptions 1. Individuals must not misrepresent their training or competence.

2. Individuals' public statements providing information about professional services and products must not contain representations or claims that are false, deceptive or misleading.

3. Individuals must not use professional or commercial affiliations in any way that would mislead or limit services to persons served professionally.

Matters of Professional Propriety 1. Individuals should announce services in a manner consonant with highest professional standards in the community.

Principle of Ethics IV

Individuals shall maintain objectivity in all matters concerning the welfare of persons served professionally.

A. Individuals who dispense products to persons served professionally shall observe the following standards:

(1) Products associated with professional practice must be dispensed to the person served as a part of a program of comprehensive habilitative care.

(2) Fees established for professional services must be independent of whether a product is dispensed.

(3) Persons served must be provided freedom of choice for the source of services and products.

(4) Price information about professional services rendered and products dispensed must be disclosed by providing to or posting for persons served a complete schedule of fees and charges in advance of rendering services, which schedule differentiates between fees for professional services and charges for products dispensed.

(5) Products dispensed to the person served must be evaluated to determine effectiveness.

Ethical Proscriptions 1. Individuals must not participate in activities that constitute a conflict of professional interest.

Matters of Professional Propriety 1. Individuals should not accept compensation for supervision or sponsorship from the clinician being supervised or sponsored.

2. Individuals should present products they have developed to their colleagues in a manner consonant with highest professional standards.

Principle of Ethics V

Individuals shall honor their responsibilities to the public, their profession, and their relationships with colleagues and members of allied professions.

Matters of Professional Propriety 1. Individuals should seek to provide and expand services to persons with speech, language and hearing handicaps as well as to assist in establishing high professional standards for such programs.

2. Individuals should educate the public about speech, language and hearing processes, speech, language and hearing problems, and matters related to professional competence.

3. Individuals should strive to increase knowledge within the profession and share research with colleagues.

4. Individuals should establish harmonious relations with colleagues and members of other professions, and endeavor to inform members of related professions of services provided by speech-language pathologists and audiologists, as well as seek information from them.

5. Individuals should assign credit to those who have contributed to a publication in proportion to their contribution.

Principle of Ethics VI

Individuals shall uphold the dignity of the profession and freely accept the profession's self-imposed standards.

A. Individuals shall inform the Ethical Practice Board of violations of this Code of Ethics.

B. Individuals shall cooperate fully with the Ethical Practice Board inquiries into matters of professional conduct related to this Code of Ethics.

Glossary of Legal Terms

Many of the terms relevant to law that were used in this book are briefly defined here. For definitions of other terms or for more complete definitions of those defined, consult the index.

Accreditation An approach used by a professional association to regulate the practice of an occupation through the establishment of standards for the curriculum and administration of programs that train new practitioners.
Administrative agency A rule-making organization created by a legislative or executive branch of government to develop, administer, and enforce the programs it has mandated in a specific subject matter area (e.g., education).
Administrative hearing A hearing conducted under the auspices of an administrative agency.
Administrative law The branch of law that deals with regulations promulgated by administrative agencies.
Advocate A person who does everything possible to insure that people receive the services that the law entitles them to receive.
Appellate courts Courts that review the decisions of trial courts when they are requested to do so.
Assault A tort resulting when someone's actions and/or words cause you to become apprehensive about being harmed by them.
Battery A tort resulting when someone intentionally touches you without your permission.
Bills Proposed laws considered by legislatures. If passed, they become statutes.
Breach of contract The failure of one or both parties to a contract to do what they agreed, or promised, to do.
Certification A voluntary mechanism by which a nongovernmental agency or association grants recognition to an individual who has met certain predetermined qualifications specified by that agency or association.
Civil law The branch of law concerned with relationships between private individuals, rather than between private individuals and society (which is the concern of criminal law).
Civil suit Litigation in which a court attempts to remedy a controversy between individuals or organizations.
Common law Legal precedent derived from court decisions.
Compensatory damages Damages intended to compensate the plaintiff for the injury he or she received from the defendant.
Complaint A document drafted by the attorney for the plaintiff in a lawsuit that indicates why the plaintiff believes he or she was legally wronged by the defendant and specifies the judicial remedy being sought.
Contract A promise or set of promises for breach of which the law gives a remedy, or the performance of which the law in some way recognizes as a duty.
Copyright The exclusive right to make and sell copies of an author's work for a limited period of time.
Corporation A business (e.g., private practice) that obtains its financing by selling stock, or shares of ownership; it is classified by the courts as a person.
Countersuit A lawsuit initiated against the plaintiff by the defendant. In a countersuit the defendant becomes the plaintiff and the plaintiff the defendant.
Criminal law The branch of law that deals with crimes, or acts against society.
Damages Money that the plaintiff is seeking from the defendant in a lawsuit to compensate for an "injury" that the plaintiff feels was done to him or her by the defendant.
Declaratory judgment A statement of clarification that a person seeks from a court regarding what the law is in a particular situation or the meaning of the law in that situation.
Defamation A tort that results from saying or writing something false and mali-

cious about someone that injures their reputation. It includes both slander and libel.
Defendant The person sued by the plaintiff in a lawsuit.
Deposition A statement made under oath in writing, ordinarily prior to a trial.
Discovery An opportunity given to each party in a lawsuit to find out prior to the trial the sorts of evidence the other party has and is likely to use at the trial.
Ex post facto laws Laws that make a crime of an act that, when it was done, was not a crime.
Expert witness A witness who both evaluates and provides evidence in his or her area of expertise.
Felonies Crimes that are not classified as misdemeanors. They usually are punishable by relatively large fines, relatively long prison sentences, and in some extremely serious cases, death.
Fraud An intentional perversion of truth for the purpose of inducing another who relies on it to part with some valuable belonging or to surrender a legal right.
Functionalism A philosophy that suggests that the decision the courts are most likely to make in a particular situation can be regarded as the law in that situation.
Informed consent Consent given by a research subject that was not obtained by coercion and did not result from the subject's failing to be fully informed about the risks involved.
Injunction An order issued by a court to a defendant to do some specific activity or to refrain from doing some specific activity.
Intentional torts Torts that result from acts that are intended to injure or harm others and/or are morally wrong.
Laws Rules that are intended to govern our interpersonal relationships; they place restrictions and obligations on our relations with others.
Libel Defamation tort resulting from false and malicious statements being communicated in written or printed form.
Licensure A legal mechanism by which a governmental agency authorizes persons who have met specified minimal standards of competency to engage in a given profession or occupation.
Licensure board A state administrative agency responsible for administering a licensure law.
Liquidated damages A specific amount of money specified in a contract that the party who breaches a contract agrees to pay to the other party in the contract.
Litigation A legal proceeding.
Lobbyist Any person who intentionally attempts to influence how legislators vote.
Malpractice Any type of negligent conduct by a professional that causes his or her patient (client) to be harmed either physically or emotionally.
Misdemeanors Relatively minor crimes that usually are punishable by relatively low fines and/or relatively short terms of imprisonment.
Natural law A philosophy suggesting that we have an obligation in our interpersonal relationships to do what is "right," "fair," "just," and "ethical."
Negligence torts Torts involving carelessness that injures or harms others (e.g., malpractice).
Nominal damages Small amounts of money that are awarded to plaintiffs when the wrong done to them did not result in an actual injury.
Partnership A business (e.g., private practice) owned by two or more persons.
Patent A grant made by the government to an inventor, conveying and securing to

him or her the exclusive right to make, use, and sell the invention for a term of years.

Plaintiff The person (or group) who initiates a lawsuit (i.e., files a complaint).

Positive law A philosophy stating that the law is what legally constituted lawmakers say it is.

Pro se litigant A defendant or plaintiff in a lawsuit who acts as his or her own attorney.

Procedural laws Laws that specify how substantive laws are to be enforced.

Property law The branch of civil law concerned with rights of ownership.

Proprietorship A business (e.g., private practice) owned by a single person.

Punitive damages Damages awarded to the plaintiff in addition to compensatory damages; their purpose is to punish the defendant.

Realism A philosophy suggesting that the unconscious prejudices judges hold are likely to influence their court decisions.

Record An account of what has been done.

Reformation A type of remedy that can be ordered by a court when a contract does not accurately reflect the agreement between the parties because of error, fraud, or ambiguous language. It is an order to revise the contract.

Registration A form of certification administered by a governmental agency in which persons who have completed the training deemed necessary by the agency to function as practitioners in a particular field have their names listed in a register (file) that is maintained by the agency.

Restitution A type of remedy that can be ordered by a court if a plaintiff has been unjustly deprived of a right or property. Restitution may or may not involve money.

Slander Defamation tort resulting from false or malicious statements being communicated in oral form.

Stare decisis The tendency of judges to base their decisions on precedent, when precedent exists, and thus not decide what already has been decided.

Statute A law passed by a legislature.

Statute of limitations A statute that specifies how long a person has after an event has occurred to initiate a suit in relation to it. A plaintiff may not be awarded the remedy sought because he or she has waited too long to initiate a suit.

Subpoena An order issued by a court to turn over certain documents to it or to testify; it is issued when a person refuses to do so voluntarily.

Substantive laws Laws that create, define, and regulate duties and rights. Such laws tell us what we should and should not do.

Summons A document that directs a person to appear in court to answer a complaint.

Torts Injuries or wrongs to individuals resulting from the dangerous or unreasonable conduct of others, that do not arise from breaching a contract, for which courts will provide a remedy by awarding compensation.

Trial courts The first courts to try, consider, or become involved with any civil or criminal case. They are at the entrance level in the hierarchies of both state and federal court systems.

Utilitarianism A philosophy that suggests that legislatures (and other lawmakers) should attempt to promote the greatest good for the greatest number of persons by making appropriate laws.

Index

Acceptance (*see* Contracts)
Accreditation, 61-65, 67-69, 74-77, 218
   American Speech-Language-Hearing Association, 74
   loss of, 75-77
   motivation for initiating, 62-65
Administration, legal aspects of, 2, 6, 140-148
   advertising, 147
   employer-employee relationship, 143-147
      governmental regulation of, 146-147
      master-servant, principal-agent, and employer-independent-contractor relationships, 143-146
      tort liability in, 145-146
   organizational structures for clinical facilities, 140-143
      corporation, 142-143, 218
      individual ownership, 141
      partnership, 141, 219
   record keeping, 147
Administrative agencies, 1, 9, 218
   hearings, 2, 3, 9, 58-60, 218
      defendants, 3
      hearing officers, 3, 58-60
      plaintiffs, 3
   regulation of services by, 2, 3
   rule making procedures, 33-34
Advertising (*see* Administration)
Advocate, serving as, 2, 3, 5, 179-180, 218
Affirmative action, 146

American Academy of Private Practice in Speech Pathology and Audiology, 148
American Board of Examiners in Speech Pathology and Audiology, 69
American Speech-Language-Hearing Association, 5, 6, 7, 9, 10, 14, 34-35, 37, 61, 65-69, 71, 73-77, 92-93, 104-106, 116, 121, 136, 146, 148, 175-177
   certificates of clinical competence, 34-35 (*see also* Certification)
Analytical positivism (*see* Law, types of: positive)
Assault (*see* Torts)

Battered children, 5
Battery (*see* Torts)
Better Business Bureau, 89
Buckley Amendment, 126

Case law (*see* Law, types of: common)
Certification, 1-2, 6, 61-67, 73-77, 218
   American Speech-Language-Hearing Association, 61-62, 73, 92
      professional ethics and, 105
   loss of, 74-77
   motivation for initiating, 62-65
   speciality, 73
Civil suits (*see* Courts)

Communication Act of 1934, 191
Communication prostheses, funding for, 42, 180
Competency, 4, 162-163
  legal definition, 86
Confidentiality, 5 (*see also* Ethics; Records, management of; Research)
Congressional Action Contact Bulletin, 178
Congressional Action Contact Network (*see* Lobbying)
Consideration (*see* Contracts)
Constitutionality, 42
Constitution of the United States, 1, 29-30, 33, 130, 174, 193-208
Consumer Product Warranties Act, 191
Contempt of court, 54
Contracts, 35-36, 78-91, 218
  breaching of, 4, 36, 41, 89, 218
  client-clinician relationship and, 2, 4, 90
  employer-employee relationships and, 145
  events that can create, 79-84
    acceptance of the offer, 82-83
    consideration exchanged, 83-84
    the offer, 80-82
  events that can interfere with creation, 84-89
    contract not in written form, 85, 88-89
    duress, 85, 88
    fraud, 85-87
    illegality, 85, 88
    incapacity, 85-86
    mistake, 85, 87-88
    offer being unconscionable, 85, 88
  implications for deaf, 86
  statute of limitations and, 42
Copyrights, 2, 5-6, 37, 129-139, 218
  Copyright Act of 1976, 131-136
    deposit and registration of the work, 135
    duration of copyright protection, 131
    material that can be copyrighted, 132-133
    notice of copyright, 135
    ownership and transfer of rights, 133
    remedies for infringement, 136
    reproduction of copyrighted material, 134-135
  objectives, 129-131
Corporation (*see* Administration)
Counteroffer, 83 (*see also* Contracts)
Courts:
  choice of in civil actions, 27-29
  civil suits, 9
  types of:
    administrative agency, 27-28
    appellate, 25-26, 51, 56, 58, 218
    claims, 27-28
    county, 26-27
    customs, 27-28
    customs and patent appeals, 27-28
    domestic relations, 26-27
    justice of the peace, 26-27
    juvenile, 26-27
    municipal, 26-27
    probate, 26-27
    small-claims, 26-27, 38
    state supreme, 26-27
    superior, 26-27
    trial, 25-26, 220
    U.S. Court of Appeals, 25, 27-28, 56
    U.S. district, 27-28
    U.S. Supreme Court, 25, 27-28, 58
Custody, 163-164

Daily Prayer of a Physician, 95-96
Damages, 218 (*see also* Lawsuits)
  for infliction of mental distress, 119
  types of:
    compensatory, 39, 218
    liquidated, 40-41, 219
    nominal, 40-41, 219
    punitive, 39-41, 220
Declaration of Helsinki, 188-190
Declaratory judgment, 40-42, 218
Defamation (*see* Torts)
Defendant, 219 (*see also* Lawsuits)
Department of Education, 32
Depositions, 51, 219
Discovery, 219 (*see also* Lawsuits)
Discrimination in hiring, 146
Due process of law, 24, 37, 53, 58, 76

Education of All Handicapped Children Act (*see* P.L. 94-142)
Equal Employment Opportunity Commission, 32
Equity, 39
Ethics, professional, 92-107
  advertising, 103-105
  AMA's Principles of Medical Ethics, 98-99, 101-103
  American Speech-Language-Hearing Association Code of Ethics, 14-15, 16, 30, 73, 81, 92-93, 95, 98, 102-106, 118, 124, 147, 173, 192, 209-215
  American Speech-Language-Hearing Association Ethical Practices Board, 106
  ASHA members who are uncertified engaging in clinical practice, 106
  CFY supervisors' responsibilities, 106
  in clinical practice, 95-104
  codes of, 1, 6-7, 10, 61, 64, 74-75, 95, 97-104
  confidentiality, 97-99
  degrees from "diploma mills," 106
  discrimination, 102-103
  dispensing of products, 105
  doing myofunctional therapy, 105

ethics of manipulation, 7
fees for clinical services provided by students, 105-106
gratuities, 106
guaranteeing improvement, 90, 104
holding paramount the welfare of persons served professionally, 96, 99, 102
honoring of contracts, 105
improvement of clinical knowledge and skills, 99-100
intersect with law and clinical practice and research, 2-8
Judeo-Christian ethics, 7
listings in telephone directories, 106
making referrals to other professionals, 96-97
monitoring compliance of others with, 102
nonspeech communication and, 106
not exploiting persons served, 101
oaths and prayers, 95-97
obligation to advance knowledge, 100
obligation to do therapy outcome research, 99
patient selection, 102-103
public statements by ASHA members, 106
relationship to law, 92-94
restraints and obligations imposed by, 1
speech-language pathologists functioning as audiologists and vice versa, 106
third-party payments, 105
truth-telling, 100-101
use of supportive personnel, 106
violation of state ethical codes, 106
Expert witness, functioning as, 2, 4, 17, 161-172, 219
in administrative hearings, 3
in competency hearings, 86
fee for serving as, 166, 171
in lawsuits, 53
projecting an appropriate image, 164-166
subjects about which speech-language pathologists and audiologists have testified, 162-164
administrative agency hearings, 164
civil court proceedings, 163-164
criminal court proceedings, 162-163
testifying, 166-171
being qualified as an expert, 167-168
cross-examination, 169-171
direct examination, 171
Ex post facto laws, 30, 219

Fair use, 134-135
Federal Food, Drug, and Cosmetic Act, 191
Federal Register, 34
Federal Trade Commission, 191-192
Felonies, 35, 219
Forms, 181-186
model release, 185
permission for participation in non-therapeutic research, 186
permission for videotaping and recording clinical work, 184
release of information, 182
request for information, 183
Fraud, 219
Freedom of Information Act, 34
Functionalism, 16, 219

Governmental Affairs Review, 74, 178
Grandfather clause, 64, 75

Hearings (*see* Administrative agencies)
Hospital, Nursing Home, Domiciliary and Medical Care Act, 192

Infliction of mental distress (*see* Torts)
Informed consent, 7, 100, 101, 120, 150-153, 155-160, 219
form for documenting, 159
Injunctions, 219 (*see also* Lawsuits)
for infliction of mental distress, 119
types of:
mandatory, 39-40
prohibitory, 39-40
Internal Revenue Service, 32, 38
Invasion of privacy (*see* Torts)
IRB: A Review of Human Subject Research, 156

Judeo-Christian tradition, 95
Judicial remedies, 39-42

Law:
intersect with professional ethics and clinical practice and research, 2-8
relevance of for the speech-language pathologist and audiologist, 1-8
types of:
administrative, 9, 218
civil, 9, 218
common, 1, 9, 16, 18, 218
constitutional, 10
criminal, 9, 218
natural, 11, 12-13, 93-94, 130, 219
positive, 14, 220
procedural, 9, 24, 37, 220
substantive, 9, 24, 37, 220
Laws, 219
categories of, 35-37
administrative, 35-36
civil, 35-37
criminal, 35
dimensions on which they vary, 10-11
enforcement of, 37-60
mechanisms used for enforcing, 9
pertaining to speech and hearing services in public schools, 11
philosophies that influence, 11-18
"conduct determined the law," 15-16

224 Index

"custom determines law's content," 13-14
"do what is fair," 12-13
"future impacts of government action should be considered in the lawmaking process," 18
"law inhibits or frustrates our instincts," 17-18
"the law is what legally constituted lawmakers say it is," 14-15
"might makes right," 12
"promote the greatest good for the greatest number," 15
"unconscious prejudices influence court decisions," 16-17
"what the courts will do with respect to a particular matter is the law," 16
precedence, 10
sources of, 18-35
 administrative agencies, 32-34
 courts, 18-29
 legislatures, 29-32
 professional organizations, 34-35
types of:
 administrative regulations, 14
 constitutional, 14
 employer's regulations, 10
 ordinances, 14
 statutes, 9-10, 14
 sunset, 10
Lawsuits, 38-58
 answering the complaint, 44, 49-50
 appeals, 56, 58
 civil, 38, 218
   steps in, 42-58
 class action, 38
 closing arguments, 55-56
 the complaint, 44-48, 218
 contingency fees in, 39
 countersuit, 38, 218
 criminal, 38
 the decision, 56-57
 defendant in, 38
 discovery, 51
 judicial remedies, 39-42
   damages, 39-41, 89
   injunctions, 39-42
 jury selection, 53-54
 motion for a directed verdict, 55
 motion for a judgment notwithstanding the verdict of the jury, 56
 motion for involuntary dismissal, 55
 opening statements, 54
 plaintiff in, 38
 pro se litigant, 38, 53, 220
 role of judge, 51-52
 role of jury, 52
 the trial, 51-58
 verdict requested:
   general, 56
   special, 56

Legal restrictions and obligations, 1
Legal system:
 impact on interpersonal relationships, 9
 overview, 9-60
Legislation, 1
 federal vs. state, 16
 natural law and, 94
Legislatures, 9
 lobbying, 173-179
 process by which bills become laws, 30-32
Libel (*see* Torts)
Licensure, 2, 6, 61-65, 69-72, 74-77, 219
 boards, 32-33, 70, 219
 individual, 70-71
 institutional, 71-72
 loss of, 1, 74-77
 motivation for initiating, 62-65
 for speech-language pathologists and audiologists, 71
Litigation, 219 (*see also* Lawsuits)
Lobbying, 2, 4-5, 29, 173-180
 approaches used, 175-178
   "bribery," 175-176
   personal discussions with legislators, 177
   preparing briefs, memorandums, legislative analyses, and draft legislation, 177-178
   testifying before legislative committees, 175-178
 ASHA Congressional Action Contact Network, 5, 174-179
 functioning as a lobbyist, 178-179
 for licensure, 70
 need for, 173-174
 role of lobbyist, 174-175, 219

Malpractice (*see* Torts)
Medicaid, 103, 105, 124
Medical Devices Amendment, 192
Medicare, 3, 5, 61, 103, 105, 124, 192
Minorities, rights of, 15
Misdemeanors, 35, 219

National Commission on Accrediting, 68
National Institute of Health, 3, 153
Negligence (*see* Torts)
Nuremberg Code, 187-188

Oath of Hippocrates, 96-98, 124
Occupational Safety and Health Administration, 146
Occupational Safety and Health Amendment of 1970, 192
Occupational Safety and Health Review Commission, 32
Offer (*see* Contracts)
Office of Education, 37
Office of Human Development, 32

Index

Partnership (*see* Administration)
Patents, 2, 5-6, 37, 129-139, 219, 220
   objectives, 129-131
   U.S. patent law, 136-138
      applying for a patent, 137-138
      notice of patent, 138
      remedies for infringement, 138
      subject matter that can be patented, 136-137
Peremptory challenges, 54
Personal injury litigation, 163
Plaintiff, 220 (*also see* Lawsuits)
Private practice, legal aspects, 2, 6, 101, 140-148 (*see also* Administration)
   functioning as an independent contractor, 145-146
   liability insurance, 116, 121
Process server, 44
Pro forma, 64-65
Property law, 35, 37, 220
Proprietorship, 220 (*see also* Administration)
Pro se litigant (*see* Lawsuits)
Public Health Service, 32
Public Law (P.L.) 94-142, 3-5, 10, 13, 15-16, 58, 161, 164, 179, 191

Realism, 17, 220
Records, management of, 2, 5, 37, 122-128
   access of clients and families to records, 125-126
   aspects on which there are legal restrictions, 123-128
   correcting errors, 126-127
   data regarded as being part of a clinic record, 123
   ownership of records, 125
   record content and documentation, 123-124
   record retention, 127
   requests for information, 127
   storage and confidentiality, 124-125
   transfer of information, 127
   use of client records for research, 127-128
Reformation, 40-41, 220
Registration, 61-65, 69-70, 72-77, 220
   loss of, 74-77
   motivation for initiating, 62-65
Rehabilitation Act of 1973, 192
Research, legal aspects of, 2, 7, 149-160
   documenting informed consent, 159-160
   need for protecting research subjects, 149, 151
   institutional committees, 149-151
   possible detrimental effects, 18
   therapeutic-nontherapeutic continuum, 153-158, 160
      mixed therapeutic-nontherapeutic clinical research, 157-158, 160
      nontherapeutic clinical research, 154-156
      therapeutic clinical research, 156-157
   use of client records for, 127-128
Respondant superior, 146
Restitution, 40-42, 89, 220
Restraint of trade, 104

Sherman Antitrust Act, 192
Slander (*see* Torts)
Social and Rehabilitation Services Program, 69
Social Security Act, 192
Social Security Administration, 3, 32, 124, 173
Stare decisis, 13, 18, 24-25, 122, 220
Statute, 220 (*see also* Laws)
Statute of limitations, 42, 220
Subpoena procedures, 5, 54, 123, 220
Suits (*see* Lawsuits)
Summons, 44, 220
Sunset laws and licensure boards, 75 (*see also* Laws)

Torts, 35-37, 108-121
   definition of, 3, 109-111, 220
   informed consent and tort litigation, 152-153
   insurance protection, 116
   intentional, 111-112, 117-120, 219
   litigation for, 3-4, 121
   negligence, 3-4, 36, 111-117, 150, 219
      contributory negligence, 115
      "reasonable man" standard, 114-115
   remedies provided by courts, 110
   response-contingent punishment and, 119-120
   statute of limitations and, 42
   strict liability, 111-112, 120, 121
   types of, 111-121
      assaults, 37, 120, 218
      battery, 37, 108, 120, 150, 152, 218
      defamation, 36-37, 118, 218
      infliction of mental distress, 37, 108, 119
      invasion of privacy, 117-118
      libel, 4, 118, 219
      malpractice, 2, 4, 39, 108-109, 116-117, 163, 219
      slander, 4, 92, 108, 117-118, 220
      trespass, 37, 108
   vs. breach of contract, 110-111
   vs. crime, 36-110
Trespass (*see* Torts)

United States Commissioner of Education, 68
United States Department of Health and Human Services, 155
United States Government Manual, 32
Utilitarianism, 15, 220

Veterans Administration, 32
Voice prints, 163

Worker's compensation, 4, 163